Marketing and Retail Pharmacy

Marketing and Retail Pharmacy

COLIN GILLIGAN
Professor of Marketing, Sheffield Business School

ROBIN LOWE
*Senior Lecturer in Marketing and
Head of the Small Business Research Unit,
Sheffield Business School*

PETER CATTEE
Managing Director, Peak Pharmacy

Supported by an educational grant from

DU PONT
PHARMA

RADCLIFFE MEDICAL PRESS

Radcliffe Medical Press Ltd
18 Marcham Road, Abingdon, Oxon OX14 1AA, UK

This book is supported by an educational grant from Du Pont Pharmaceuticals Ltd. The information and views expressed in this book are those of the authors and are not necessarily those of Du Pont Pharmaceuticals Ltd.

British Library Cataloguing in Publication Data

A catalogue record for this book is available from the British Library.

ISBN 1 85775 202 3

Library of Congress Cataloging-in-Publication Data is available.

Typeset by Advance Typesetting Ltd, Oxon

Contents

The authors

Colin Gilligan is Professor of Marketing at Sheffield Business School. He is the author of books on advertising, business decision making, international marketing, marketing for the professions and strategic marketing management and, most recently, strategic planning. Over the past ten years, he has acted as a consultant to a wide variety of organizations, including numerous professional practices.

Robin Lowe is Senior Lecturer in Marketing and Head of the Small Business Research Unit at Sheffield Business School. He has 25 years experience in management and consultancy in both large and small organizations. He is the author of books on international marketing and, with Colin Gilligan, marketing for the professions.

Peter Cattee is the founder and Managing Director of Peak Pharmacy. Established in 1981, it is one of the largest medium-sized independent regional pharmacy chains in the country with, at the time of writing, more than 30 branches.

In 1997, the British Association of Medical Managers awarded Gilligan C and Lowe R *Marketing and Health Care Organizations* (Radcliffe Medical Press, Oxford) the title *The 1997 Medical Management Book of the Year.*

Preface

This short book, which is based upon our experiences of working with a wide variety of retail pharmacies, is designed to provide pharmacists with a clear understanding of the nature of marketing and of the ways in which it might possibly contribute to the effective management of their businesses as we move towards the 21st century. In designing the book, we have concentrated on producing short(ish) chapters that are capable not only of being digested easily in one sitting but which, through a series of questions and checklists, may readily be applied to a business.

In working your way through the book and its various checklists, you should not, however, focus only upon the individual questions that we pose, but should also spend time trying to identify the underlying picture that emerges. Is it the case, for example, that you *really* recognize the nature and significance of the changes taking place and have a strategy for coming to terms with them, or is it that there is a lack of any real strategy, and that you are wedded to past and increasingly inappropriate approaches?

Having reached the end of the book, you should have a far clearer idea not only of the nature and purpose of marketing, but also of the ways in which the business can best make use of marketing techniques and, by means of a series of action plans, move ahead to make the most of the undoubted opportunities that exist.

If you feel sufficiently inspired to go further in your study of marketing, you might turn to: *Strategic Marketing Management: planning, implementation and control* by Professors Dick Wilson and Colin Gilligan (published by Butterworth Heinemann in 1997).

Colin Gilligan
Robin Lowe
Peter Cattee
June 1997

Dedication

This book is dedicated to the authors' wives, Rosie, Sylvia and Jane, and children, Ben Gilligan, Jonathan and Catherine Lowe, and Thomas, Joseph and Alice Cattee, for their support; and to the pharmacists whose marketing programme, it is hoped, will benefit from the book.

The challenges facing pharmacies

Having read this chapter, you should:

- understand the nature and significance of the challenges facing pharmacies

- have a better understanding of the factors that contribute to good pharmacy management

- have gained an insight into the quality of the management within your pharmacy.

The need for a more conscious, focused and proactive approach to the management of pharmacies has increased substantially over the last few years. Because of this, we begin this book not by plunging straight into a detailed discussion of the marketing process, but by taking a broader approach in which we highlight some of the challenges that pharmacists are now having to face. Having done this, we move on to examine some of the characteristics of good and bad management practice. It is against this background that, in subsequent chapters, we turn our attention to the question of marketing and how it might best contribute to the management of pharmacies as we move towards the 21st century.

THE CHALLENGES FACING PHARMACISTS

As the first step, refer to Box 1.1 and begin by identifying the six principal challenges that you believe your pharmacy is likely to face

---

Box 1.1:   The short- and long-term challenges being faced by the pharmacy

The six principal challenges that the pharmacy is likely to face in the short term and the long term are:

Short term challenges

1. . . . .

2. . . . .

3. . . . .

4. . . . .

5. . . . .

6. . . . .

Long-term challenges

1. . . . .

2. . . . .

3. . . . .

4. . . . .

5. . . . .

6. . . . .

---

and have to come to terms with in the short term (i.e. the next 12 to 18 months) and then the longer term.

Although the particular challenges faced will quite obviously vary – possibly significantly – from one pharmacy to another, our work with different pharmacies over the past three years has identified a number of areas that pharmacists see as being of particular concern. These include:

- dealing with two separate areas of business: the NHS prescription part which typically contributes around 80% of the revenue and the counter sales which contribute 20%.

In the prescription business:

- dependence upon one source of income

- the problem of the customers being split from the payers (the NHS)
- the pressure on health spending
- the continual erosion of the margin for dispensing, now down to around 17%
- the negotiating strength and increased ambition of the large pharmacy chains
- the increased concentration of retailing generally, leading to the supermarket chains seeking opportunities in the pharmacy sector
- the fragmentation of the pharmacy market
- the geographic context
- the importance of the right location in relation to GP surgeries
- prescription charges
- increasing drug costs.

For the counter sales

- changing shopping patterns with customers increasingly purchasing from supermarkets and the resulting slippage in the customer base of local pharmacies
- the more frequent challenges to the resale price maintenance agreement by the multiple retailers
- an ageing population
- more knowledgeable and demanding customers with greater expectations of pharmacists and their staff, together with a willingness to complain
- a greater accountability to seemingly ever more demanding health authorities
- increased choice for customers
- a need to decide more clearly upon the focus of the pharmacy and, in particular, to decide which existing and new services to concentrate on
- greater financial pressures

- a need for more attention to be paid to the pharmacy's image
- the need for pharmacies to develop more effective, and possibly more mature relationships with general practices, nursing homes and others
- a need for increased and improved staff training and motivation
- an increase in the volume of paperwork
- computerization and data protection
- increased crime and customer aggression and its effect upon pharmacy staff
- the need for a more competitive philosophy
- setting and meeting targets
- the need for better internal and external communication
- the management of the relationship between the pharmacists and the other members of the pharmacy staff
- issues of quality.

Although this is not an exhaustive list and, as we comment above, the relative importance of each of the points is likely to vary greatly from one pharmacy to another, it highlights the nature and breadth of the changes and challenges that are currently facing pharmacies and with which the pharmacy management team needs to come to terms. For your viewpoint as a pharmacist, the question that must be considered, of course, is how best each of these challenges can be managed. However, before trying to answer this, consider the questions in Box 1.2 and then ask yourself what message is beginning to emerge. Is it the case, for example, that the pharmacy's management, whether a single individual or a team, not only recognizes the nature and significance of the current and emerging challenges but has begun to come to terms with them by means of a deliberate and strategic approach to the management of the pharmacy, or is it that there is a general reluctance to change old habits and working practices?

Box 1.2: Following on from the answers that you gave to the questions in Box 1.1:

1. To what extent have these challenges been given *explicit* recognition?

2. What *specific* plans exist to deal with them?

3. Has the *responsibility* for dealing with these challenges been clearly allocated?

THE CHARACTERISTICS OF GOOD AND BAD MANAGEMENT

Over the past 50 years, a considerable amount has been written about the characteristics of good and bad management. One result of this is that a series of initially general, but now increasingly specific, guidelines exist. However, before looking at some of these, consider the question in Box 1.3.

Box 1.3: The characteristics of good and bad management

What do you consider to be the six principal characteristics of good and bad management?

The characteristics of good management are:	The characteristics of bad management are:
1.	1. ....
2.	2. ....
3.	3. ....
4.	4. ....
5.	5. ....
6.	6. ....

The reality, of course, is that it is difficult (if not impossible) to identify the six or ten characteristics of good and bad management that will apply equally to every type and size of organization. What we can do, however, is to identify the sorts of area to which every organization, be it a pharmacy or a multinational manufacturer of foodstuffs or cars, needs to give serious consideration. Included within these are:

- a statement of the organization's mission and overall purpose

- the development of strong and positive values that are understood and adhered to by all staff and which the senior management are not prepared to compromise

- the development of clear and realistic objectives which, where possible, are agreed as the results of discussions amongst the staff so that there is a sense of shared ownership of the goals and strategy

- strong and unambiguous patterns of communication that allow information to go upwards, downwards and sideways quickly without being distorted

- a sense of teamwork

- a clear allocation of responsibility

- well-defined boundaries of authority that maintain control without unnecessarily stifling creativity

- a sustained effort to motivate staff at all levels

- systems for monitoring progress and feeding back the results, which then lead to corrective action being taken

- a climate that encourages rather than suppresses ideas

- a management philosophy that encourages a degree of independence amongst staff

- a management philosophy that encourages staff to get things done correctly and on time

- someone who takes responsibility for driving the strategy

- a recognition of staff needs (both personal and organizational)

- a willingness to experiment

and, most important of all

- an open and consistent management style, since one of the most widely accepted findings in management research is that one of the prime demotivators of staff is a lack of management consistency. Where the approach adopted fluctuates between autocratic, democratic and *laissez-faire* styles, seemingly depending upon how the wind is blowing, staff end up being confused and tend to focus upon a series of increasingly short-term issues.

Taking each of these areas in turn, first compare them with the list of characteristics of good management that you developed for Box 1.3 and, second, consider how well (or how badly) your pharmacy is doing.

These ideas have also been brought together in the powerful and widely used 7-S framework, which was developed in the USA in the 1980s by the management consultants, McKinsey (Figure 1.1).

The importance of the first three elements – strategy, structure and systems – has long been recognized and they are considered to be the **hardware** of successful management. The other four – style, staff, skills and shared values – are the **software**.

For much of the past 50 years, management thinking has been firmly based on the need for ensuring that the hardware elements exist. Thus, a successful organization, it has been argued, builds on a **strategy** to achieve its goals, develops an appropriate organizational **structure** and then equips the organization with the sorts of information, planning, control and reward **systems** needed to ensure that the job gets done. The starting point in this thinking is therefore that a strategy is needed before decisions on structure and systems are made.

The importance of the four software elements has been given substantially increased recognition over the past decade, largely as a result of research work in what came to be labelled 'excellent' companies; these were organizations that achieved substantially better levels of performance and customer/patient satisfaction than their competitors. The characteristics of these four software elements are:

Style:
Employees share a broadly common way of thinking and behaving. In organizations such as Marks & Spencer and McDonald's, for example, all employees are taught to smile at customers and treat them in a particular and caring way.

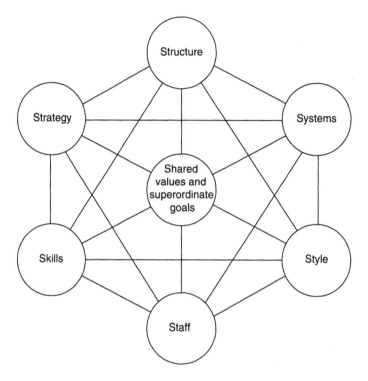

Figure 1.1:   The McKinsey 7-S framework

Skills:
Employees are fully trained in the sorts of skills that are needed to carry out the strategy.

Staff:
The people recruited are capable, well trained and given the jobs that will best allow them to make use of their talents.

Shared values:
The employees share the same values and understand where the organization is going and what it stands for.

Given these comments consider how your pharmacy performs in relation to each of these dimensions; the framework for this appears in Box 1.4.

Box 1.4: Applying the McKinsey 7-S framework to your pharmacy

1. Looking at each of the elements of the 7-S framework, how does your pharmacy score? (1 = very poor, 5 = very good)

	Score 1–5
Strategy	＿＿＿
Structure	＿＿＿
Systems	＿＿＿
Style	＿＿＿
Skills	＿＿＿
Staff	＿＿＿
Shared values	＿＿＿
Total	＿＿＿

2. Where are the areas of greatest weakness?

3. What scope exists for improvement?

4. What are you planning to do about this?

With regard to the software elements, the most important single factor is arguably the idea of shared values. There are several ways in which shared values can be developed within a pharmacy, in particular by means of an open management style that encourages discussion, communication and a sense of common purpose amongst all staff. Between you, you should therefore aim for a statement that brings together the *core values* of the pharmacy (for example, a fundamental commitment to quality and excellence which, irrespective of the circumstances, you are not willing to compromise), and a *vision* of the sort of pharmacy that, as a team, you are trying to create. Having done this, there must then be a commitment to these values that is *consistently* reflected in the behaviour of the pharmacy team. Without this it is almost inevitable that the staff will all too quickly recognize that little more than lip service is being paid to these ideas, with the result that their commitment to these values will quickly disappear.

SUMMARY

Within this chapter, we have identified a number of the challenges that pharmacies are currently having to face and highlighted some of the principal characteristics of good and bad management. In the light of your answers to the questions that we have posed, consider the following:

1.   What underlying picture of the pharmacy emerges?

2.   What do you feel are the principal causes of this picture, be it good or bad?

3.   What answers do you feel that the staff within the pharmacy might have given to the questions posed in Boxes 1.1–1.4? To what extent do these differ from your views? What are the reasons for and implications of this?

So what is marketing?

Having read this chapter, you should:

- understand the marketing concept and how it can be applied within a pharmacy

- appreciate the significance of different stakeholder groups and the need to take their expectations into account

- understand the structure of the marketing process

- appreciate the significance of the need for a distinct competitive stance.

Given the nature of our comments in Chapter 1, it is apparent that with pharmacies currently facing some of their biggest changes and challenges of the post-war period, the need for tighter, more professional and forward-looking management is now greater than ever before. In many cases this has meant a substantial rethink of how pharmacies are run and how a variety of the managerial tools and techniques that were seen previously to be the prerogative of manufacturers or the multiple retailers, might now possibly contribute to the better and more effective management of their pharmacies. Prominent amongst these is the whole area of marketing. In many cases, however, there appears still to be a fundamental misunderstanding amongst pharmacists of precisely what marketing involves and how it might most realistically contribute, either to the effective day-to-day management of the pharmacy, or indeed to its longer-term development.

In this chapter, we concentrate on overcoming some of the more common preconceptions and misconceptions that we have come across in our discussions with pharmacists and move towards developing a framework that should go some way towards establishing a stronger – and far more effective – marketing and patient-centred orientation within the pharmacy.

WHAT MARKETING IS AND WHAT MARKETING IS NOT

As a starting point, consider the four statements in Box 2.1 to see which corresponds most closely with your view of marketing.

Box 2.1:   Marketing is ...

1.   ... the same as advertising

2.   ... something that is used solely by manufacturing and large retailing organizations and is of little or no real relevance to pharmacists

3.   ... manipulative and a disguised approach to a hard sell

4.   ... an approach to management that applies to all types of organization, since it puts the customer at the very centre of the operation and directs resources in such a way that the customer achieves a high(er) level of satisfaction in a cost-effective manner.

Those of you who answered 'yes' to any, or indeed all, of the first three should go to the bottom of the class. Those who agreed with number four get top marks.

So what then is wrong with the first three statements? In the case of the first of these, we can illustrate its limitations by focusing upon examples of large organizations with whose activities you will undoubtedly be familiar, and which have developed a strong reputation for consistently effective marketing and high levels of customer satisfaction. If we ask members of the public to identify three or four examples of the sort of organization that they consider to be good at marketing, the same names almost invariably crop up. Prominent amongst these are Coca Cola, McDonald's, Marks & Spencer and The Body Shop. In the case of Coca Cola and McDonald's, both companies concentrate upon using substantial amounts of advertising to communicate clear and simple messages ('Things go better with Coke' and 'There's nothing quite like a McDonald's'), which are understood and meaningful to customers across the world. They market consistently reliable products and provide levels of service that rarely disappoint. Marks & Spencer, by contrast, has achieved a similarly strong position with little or no advertising, whilst The Body Shop is successful despite spending very little on advertising, packaging or store layout. Marketing and advertising are not, therefore, one and the same thing. Rather, advertising is just one of the marketing tools available.

The third common misconception is that marketing is almost invariably manipulative and is quite simply hard selling in disguise; timeshare holiday companies are a notorious example of this. In the long term, however, customer satisfaction cannot be built on manipulation or false promises. Customers may fall victim to it the first time, but only rarely on a second occasion. In the case of timeshare, most members of the public − not just those who have fallen foul of the timeshare touts − are now only too aware of the exaggerated offers that they typically make and are suspicious of almost any offer that is made, regardless of how attractive it appears. The unfortunate result of this has, of course, been that the reputable companies in the industry (and yes, they do exist), which offer a worthwhile product, have also been affected. Because of this, the opportunity for the market to be developed to its full potential has been lost − probably for ever − not necessarily because of any failure of the product or service offered, but because of the unacceptably high-pressure selling techniques that have been used.

Given these examples, we should be in a far clearer position to identify what marketing in its truest sense means and what it involves. Although it is difficult to list all of the activities that are typically covered by marketing, the most important can be identified as:

- monitoring the external environment (what is happening outside the organization and over which it has no control), with a view to identifying opportunities and threats

- contributing to the discussion about the nature of and direction that the organization should pursue and the competitive stance that should be adopted

- determining the range of products or services that should be offered

- influencing the levels of customer satisfaction that are to be aimed for

- deciding upon the image that is to be projected

- managing the elements of the marketing mix on a day-to-day basis (the make-up of the mix is discussed at a later stage in this chapter)

- developing and implementing a system of feedback and control that is capable of providing a clear picture of just how well the organization is performing.

It follows from this that the essence of good marketing in all organizations, including pharmacies, involves both a strong *external* and a clear *internal* orientation. External in that we are concerned with building a clear picture of what is currently happening and what is likely to happen in the future outside the organization, so that we might identify and capitalize on any opportunities that exist and take action to avoid or minimize the impact of any threats; and internal in terms of making sure that what we offer and intend doing is appropriate and feasible and that the staff understand and are fully committed to this.

DEFINITIONS OF MARKETING

It should be apparent from what has been said so far that marketing is a much more complex activity than simply selling or advertising the product or service that the organization, be it Marks & Spencer or a pharmacy, has decided to provide, something that is reflected in the numerous definitions of marketing that exist; Box 2.2 shows just a small selection of these.

Whilst you might feel that some changes in the definition are needed to reflect the specifics of your own pharmacy's situation, the core elements of **analysis**, **anticipation** and **meeting the requirements of customers** are fundamental. It is for this reason that, for us, the most meaningful definition of marketing is:

- Marketing is all about developing a really meaningful competitive advantage, and then exploiting it to the full.

Box 2.2: Definitions of marketing

- Marketing is the management process for identifying, anticipating and satisfying customers' requirements profitably (Chartered Institute of Marketing).

- Marketing is the central dimension of any business. It is the whole business seen from the point of view of its final result, that is, from the customers' point of view (Peter Drucker).

- Marketing is all about customer satisfaction and moving heaven and earth to achieve this more effectively than other organizations (Anon).

- The marketing concept represents an 'outside-in' view of the organization, in that a deliberate attempt is made to look at the organization and its products and services from the viewpoint of the customer. In doing this, a far greater emphasis is placed upon meeting customers' needs, emphasizing the product's benefits, achieving higher levels of internal co-ordination and generally achieving a far better match between what the customer needs and what the organization provides (Colin Gilligan and Robin Lowe).

In making this comment, we have several thoughts in mind. Perhaps the most obvious is that if your pharmacy does not have a clearly developed and (meaningful) competitive advantage or strong selling proposition, there is no reason why a prospective customer should come to you rather than a competitor. However, having developed a competitive advantage you need then to exploit it to the full.

SO WHAT IS A COMPETITIVE ADVANTAGE? ESTABLISHING THE COMPETITIVE STANCE

At its most basic, a competitive advantage is anything that you are capable of doing more effectively than another pharmacy. However, in many cases the sorts of things that organizations view as a competitive advantage are perceived by customers to be of little real significance. In thinking about competitive advantage, you should

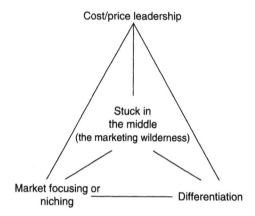

Cost/price leadership

Stuck in
the middle
(the marketing wilderness)

Market focusing or
niching   Differentiation

Figure 2.1:   The competitive stance

therefore focus upon the possible bases for differentiating your pharmacy from its competitors in a way that customers will see to be of value *to them*. All too often, however, pharmacies end up doing broadly the same thing and projecting an image that is essentially the same as every other pharmacy in the locality.

To help in the process of developing a competitive advantage and a distinct (and distinctive) competitive stance, Figure 2.1 provides a useful starting point. The thinking behind the diagram is straightforward and reflects the idea that there are, in essence, only three possible generic competitive strategies:

- a cost/price-based strategy
- market focusing or niching
- a differentiated approach.

A cost/price-based strategy is exactly what the words suggest and reflects four beliefs:

1. that low prices are the most important single influence upon the customer's choice of pharmacy

2. that the 'low price' message can be communicated to the market

3. that a price-based strategy is sustainable
4. that it will prove profitable.

By contrast, a market nicher focuses upon often highly specific areas of customer need and then concentrates upon building a reputation as one of the few specialists in this area; for example as a specialist in providing aids to help people who are disabled, or particular types of health or beauty treatment.

The third competitive strategy – differentiation – is based on the idea that customers are not necessarily primarily motivated by cost and do not have a highly specific need. Instead, they are attracted by a package of factors such as the pharmacy's breadth and depth of products, its size, the location, its general reputation, and so on. It is the unique combination of these that enables the pharmacy to achieve a differentiated position.

In many cases, however, the choice of strategy is either inappropriate for the market or is pursued with insufficient clarity (in other words, the market fails to understand the message and does not perceive the pharmacy in the way intended). The result is a confused market position in which the pharmacy ends up stuck in the middle with no obvious distinguishing characteristics. In these circumstances, there is no real reason why a prospective customer should choose one pharmacy rather than another. The reality, of course, is that many pharmacies, particularly in the provinces, find themselves in this 'stuck in the middle' position. As generalists, they have few opportunities to differentiate themselves from their competitors in the same street or town, apart from the least attractive form of competition – low prices.

Recognizing this and the importance of a clear and sustainable competitive stance, consider the following questions:

1. What is the current primary element of your competitive strategy? (Where do you appear in Figure 2.1?)
2. How are your competitors competing?
3. What image do you currently have?
4. What areas of specialism exist within the pharmacy?
5. What scope do they offer as a basis for a more proactive strategy?
6. What areas of market need exist? In what ways might they be reflected in a more obvious competitive strategy?

THE TWO LEVELS OF MARKETING

If marketing is to make a significant contribution to a pharmacy, it needs to operate at two levels. At its most fundamental it represents the development of a clear and appropriate competitive stance and the pursuit of an underlying philosophy of customer satisfaction that should guide everything that the pharmacists, pharmacy technicians and counter staff do. On a day-to-day level, it is concerned with issues such as the specifics of the service that is offered, the image that is projected, and how and where the service is to be presented. The essence of marketing is therefore to get everyone to pull together and work towards the common goal of customer/patient satisfaction. If this is done, and done effectively, the benefits can be considerable and include:

- higher levels of customer satisfaction
- a far greater likelihood of identifying market opportunities in their early stages
- a higher level of awareness of those factors that will ultimately prove to be a threat
- a better sense of direction and co-ordination
- a greater opportunity for staff to take more responsibility without loss of control
- higher levels of staff motivation as a result of their greater understanding, involvement, responsibility and commitment.

THE MARKETING PROCESS

In the light of our comments so far, we can identify the principal strands of a marketing programme as being concerned with the development of a clear understanding of three distinct elements:

1. the pressures of the environment (and hence the nature of any opportunities and threats that currently exist and which are likely to emerge in the future)

2. the demands, needs or expectations of customers and how these are likely to change

3. what the pharmacy is really capable of delivering.

It follows from this that the marketing process consists of four stages:

1. analysis

2. planning

3. evaluation and implementation

4. feedback and control.

These are illustrated in Figure 2.2 and expanded in Box 2.3.

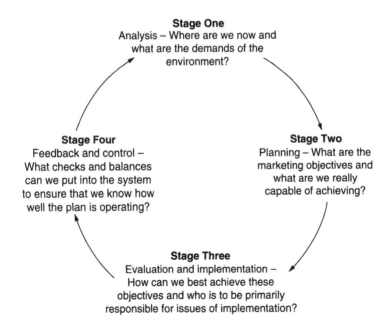

Figure 2.2: The marketing process

Box 2.3:   The four stages of the marketing process

Stage One: Analysis (Where are we now?)
Analysing and understanding:

- the environment

- the customers' and other stakeholders' needs and expectations

- the competition (what other pharmacies are doing and what we can learn from them and improve upon).

Stage Two: Planning (Where do we want to go?)
Planning for action by:

- researching customers' current and future needs

- setting objectives and standards

- evaluating the pharmacy's capabilities

- planning for change.

Stage Three: Evaluation and implementation (How might we get there?)
Implementing the plan by:

- managing the marketing mix

- marketing the plan internally

- developing stakeholder relationships.

Stage Four: Feedback and control (How can we check how well the plan is operating?)
Controlling the plan by:

- developing checks and balances

- monitoring progress

- taking corrective action.

Stage One: Market analysis

The first of these four stages involves developing a clear understanding of the variety of factors outside the pharmacy that for the most part cannot be controlled but which determine how the pharmacy operates and which are capable of having a very real influence upon performance. Included within this are the general environment, the changing needs of customers and other stakeholders, and the behaviour of competitors.

Stage Two: Marketing planning

Against the background of what emerges from the market analysis, the emphasis then needs to shift to planning and, in particular, to the identification of the goals, objectives and standards that the pharmacy will pursue. In doing this, detailed consideration needs to be given to an assessment of the pharmacy's true capabilities, since these determine how likely it is that objectives will be met and whether any gaps exist between the pharmacy's aspirations, objectives and its capabilities (in other words, what you are really capable of delivering). This information can then be brought together in the form of a plan that will be the blueprint for development.

Stage Three: Evaluating and implementing the idea

Following this, the focus turns to the question of how to implement the plan. It has long been recognized that the implementation stage is typically the most difficult part of the marketing planning process, since it is only too easy to lose sight of the objectives, to be blown off course by unforeseen events, and to become preoccupied with day-to-day pressures, with the result that longer-term issues are ignored. A key element of marketing is therefore concerned with the question of how best to manage the available resources in as effective a manner as possible and ensure that the objectives that have been set are achieved. Because the largest and most costly resource in pharmacies is the staff, much of the implementation phase is, of necessity, concerned with mobilizing the staff and other stakeholders, including those who supply the pharmacy with services and products, by making sure that they fully understand what is expected of them and that they then contribute in the most appropriate way.

However, as well as with staff, implementation is integrally tied up with how well the marketing mix is managed. Although we discuss the marketing mix in detail in Chapter 8 , there are several comments that can usefully be made at this stage. The marketing mix, which consists of the seven elements illustrated in Figures 2.3 and 2.4, and is sometimes referred to as the 7Ps, represents the marketing man

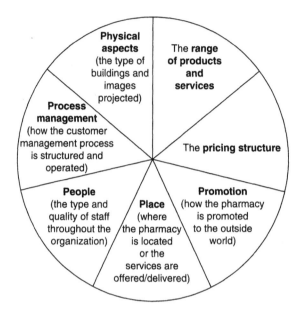

Figure 2.3:   The seven elements of the marketing mix

or woman's tool kit and is made up of the various elements that,
despite the strict guidelines and controls that exist within pharmacies,
can be *managed* in order to shape the profile of the pharmacy that
is presented to the world. As such, the appropriateness of the mix
(i.e. the match between the mix and the demands of the environment) has a direct influence upon the pharmacy's performance.

Stage Four: Feedback and control

Having implemented the marketing plan, attention needs then to be
paid to measuring the performance levels that are being achieved
with a view to identifying where scope exists for modification and
improvement. There is, therefore, a need to monitor performance
under a variety of headings. These might include:

• financial performance, including income, expenditure and
profitability

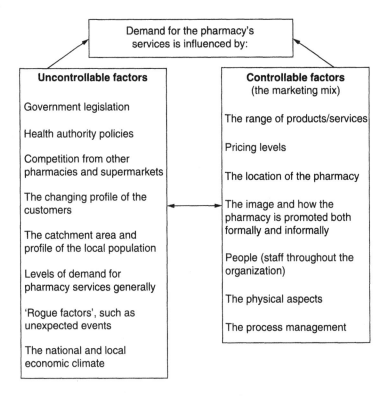

Figure 2.4:   The marketing mix and the medical environment

- relative competitive performance (how well or badly has the pharmacy performed in relation to those pharmacies that are seen to be direct competitors)

- the pharmacist's level of commitment and performance, including the work undertaken, external posts and personal development

- staff performance, including turnover, attitudes, absenteeism, motivation, development and training

- customer management, including the demand for services, levels of satisfaction with the pharmacy and customers lost to competitors

- premises management, including the nature and suitability of any improvements made

- communications management, including the development of the pharmacy's image and the success of any promotional initiatives
- the general publicity of the pharmacy
- the development of new services
- the introduction of new or modified systems for dealing with prescriptions.

However, if this is to be a meaningful activity, it presupposes that the objectives that were set in Stage Two have been clearly set and provide a sound basis for measure or comparison over time; this is an issue to which we will return in later chapters.

Box 2.4:   Deciding upon the focus

David Pearson is a 32-year old who has recently bought a shop with contract permission in a village of 3200 people. The premises are next to the local post office. He has never run his own business before and is learning as he goes along. The rent and rates on the premises are £6500, whilst the stock, valued at £27 000, has been financed with an extended credit deal from wholesalers. At the moment he is trying to decide on the focus of the business and, in particular, whether to take a largely commercial or a health care message.

What would you suggest should be taken into account in deciding upon this?

SUMMARY

Within this chapter, we have focused on the nature of marketing and the marketing process as well as on the ways in which marketing is capable of being applied within pharmacies. Although a marketing programme needs to reflect, or at least take account of, the expectations of various stakeholder groups, the primary focus is on how best to develop a truly customer-oriented pharmacy. It is this issue that is developed in the next chapter.

3

Developing the customer-centred pharmacy: the first few steps

Having read this chapter, you should:

- understand the dimensions of a customer-centred pharmacy
- appreciate the significance of the differences between features and benefits
- have a clearer insight to the benefits that your pharmacy currently offers and is capable of offering in the future
- understand in greater detail what it is that your customers want from the pharmacy.

In order to develop a market-oriented and truly customer-centred pharmacy, there is an obvious need to understand in detail your market for pharmacy products and services and, in particular, the sorts of factors that are likely to lead to higher levels of customer satisfaction. Without this information, any marketing effort will be unfocused and, at best, of only limited value. So what is it that contributes to customer satisfaction? Although most pharmacists would argue that they have a clear idea of this, it is only the customers themselves who are really able to answer the question.

Whenever we begin a consultancy assignment, we pose a deceptively simple question: what *benefits* are your customers really looking for? The significance of this is that people only rarely, if ever, buy a product or service for its own sake. Instead, they buy it for the benefits that it provides. Perhaps the most commonly cited example of this is the purchase of a drill, which, as the American management guru, Theodore Levitt, pointed out in the 1950s, is bought not for its physical qualities but in order to provide holes. It follows from this that a manufacturer of twist drills will eventually go out of business if a laser can do the job twice as accurately, twice as fast and at half the cost.

By the same token, cars such as Porsche, Mercedes, BMW and Jaguar, whether we like to admit it or not, are bought as much for their status, image and prestige as anything else. We then justify the purchase by highlighting features such as the build quality, the glacier-like depreciation, the pre- and after-sales services, reliability, and so on. By the same token, research in the expensive boxed chocolates market reveals that the buying motives are only rarely concerned with taste, but are instead more commonly to do with the perceived value of the product as a gift. In the case of the beer market, the primary buying motives amongst the 18–22 year olds have consistently been shown to be concerned not with the beer's taste or strength, but with the images associated with the brand and peer group pressure.

Recognition of this highlights the need for a clear and detailed understanding of the distinctions that exist between features and benefits, since it is this understanding that underpins any attempt to develop a truly customer-centred pharmacy. It is, for example, only too easy to talk about the things that pharmacists do (the features) rather than what customers get from them (the benefits). The way in which this is typically manifested is in terms of how a pharmacist solves a customer's problem. The application of the pharmacist's skills is the feature. However, looking at it from the customers' point of view, they go to a pharmacist with a problem that needs to be solved. The extent to which this is achieved is influenced only partly by the skills that the pharmacist uses and the products the pharmacist supplies. The other part of the solution consists of a series of non-pharmacy elements that are normally referred to as customer care (this typically includes the counter and dispensary staff, and the general customer management process). If these non-pharmacy elements fail to work effectively, customers may well go away having been provided with a solution to the problem but feeling unhappy, unconvinced by their overall treatment in the pharmacy and generally dissatisfied. This creates the paradoxical situation in which the highest possible level of pharmacy skills have been used to obtain an excellent result, yet the customer may be unaware of this, having judged the performance of the pharmacy on the tangible non-pharmacy elements of the service. Examples of this might include lengthy waiting times for a prescription to be prepared (possibly the next day if the drug is not available), a poor range of non-prescription products or nowhere provided for a confidential conversation with the pharmacist.

COMING TO TERMS WITH THE BENEFITS

In order to understand more fully the benefits that the pharmacy currently offers, you need to begin by looking at features from the viewpoint of the customer. There are several ways of doing this, although perhaps the most useful is by focusing in turn upon each of the seven principal elements of the marketing mix. Although the detail of the mix is discussed at a later stage in Chapter 8, we identified its components in Chapter 2 and can illustrate the features/benefit distinction here by focusing upon just one of these dimensions, that of the product or service.

The cornerstone of any marketing programme is the nature of the product or service offered, since virtually all other marketing elements and decisions are directly influenced by this. In the case of pharmacies, the product/service is the collection of benefits that the customer desires. At the core of this 'product' are the pharmacy services in which the traditional issues of excellence, quality and expertise are paramount; examples of those that are typically offered appear in Box 3.1.

Surrounding these core pharmacy services are the various support services, including the outer appearance of the pharmacy, the manner in which the staff greet and attend to customers, the speed

---

Box 3.1:   **The core pharmacy services**

- Fulfilling prescriptions accurately.

- Ensuring that the patient is reminded of the dosage rates, by providing a clear and legible label.

- Providing pharmacy only (P) drugs and explaining how they should be taken and any specific side effects.

- Having a good range of over the counter (OTC) or GSL (General sales list) treatments available.

with which prescriptions are dealt, the help that counter staff and the pharmacists can provide and the empathy that staff can build up with their customers, including local general practices and nursing homes.

Although the question of what benefits the pharmacy currently offers and what it is capable of developing is considered in far greater detail in Chapter 8, a useful first step at this stage is to begin by thinking about the nature and significance of the benefits that customers derive from the services that are offered. In doing this, Herzberg's two-factor theory of motivation can be of some help. The theory distinguishes between **satisfiers** (factors that create satisfaction) and **dissatisfiers** (factors that create dissatisfaction). In the case of a car, for example, the absence of a warranty would be a dissatisfier. The existence of a warranty, however, is not a satisfier since it is not one of the principal reasons for buying a car; as we commented at an earlier stage, these are more likely to be the car's looks, its performance and the status the driver feels that it confers.

There are several implications of this theory for the marketing of pharmacies, the two most significant of which are, first, that the seller (i.e. the pharmacist) needs to be fully aware of the dissatisfiers that, while they will not by themselves sell the product, can easily 'unsell' it. (For example, customers soon tire of being routinely kept waiting for prescriptions or having to call back later for a frequently used drug, and general practitioners and customers get fed up with waiting if the telephone is not answered promptly.) The second implication, that follows logically from this, is that all pharmacy staff need to understand in detail the various satisfiers and then concentrate on not only supplying them, but also giving emphasis to them, so that customers are fully aware of them.

It should be apparent from this that achieving a truly customer-centred pharmacy is a potentially difficult task and, for most pharmacies, is likely to involve significant changes in operating practice and culture. Recognizing this, consider the following questions and then move on to the checklist that appears in Box 3.2.

- What are the principal satisfiers and dissatisfiers within the pharmacy?

- What are we doing/can we do to increase the satisfiers and reduce or completely abolish the dissatisfiers?

Box 3.2:   How serious are we about customer satisfaction?

Marks out of ten

- 1 = Very poor performance
- 5 = Average performance, but possibly with considerable scope for improvement
- 10 = Excellent performance

How good are we at: **Score**

1. Measuring levels of customer satisfaction?   _____

2. Using measures of customer satisfaction to change the pharmacy's policies and operating procedures?   _____

3. Using customer satisfaction measures to
    - evaluate staff
    - reward staff?   _____

4. Ensuring that *all* staff have a clear understanding of our policy on customer care and quality?   _____

5. Setting measurable goals for levels of customer care and quality?   _____

6. Discussing with staff the customers' needs and expectations?   _____

7. Taking formal note of what staff say about customers' needs and expectations and the extent to which they are being met?   _____

8. Setting a good example as pharmacists of the levels of service and quality that we say are important?   _____

9. Providing opportunities for staff to work together to overcome obstacles in order to achieve high(er) levels of quality and service?   _____

10. Evaluating how other pharmacies operate and the standards that they are achieving?   _____

11. Evaluating what organizations outside the pharmacy profession do, with a view to learning from them?   _____

continued

Box 3.2: *continued*

12. Implementing a clearly stated and realistic policy
    on customer service and quality?   _____

                              Total score (out of 120)   _____

The scoring process

You should work through the 12 questions in order to arrive at a score. The scores are than aggregated and averaged. The overall measures of commitment to customer service and satisfaction can then be assessed against the following scale:

With a score of 59 or less, questions can be asked about the pharmacy's commitment to customer care. Fundamental changes are needed, both in the pharmacy's philosophy and organizational structure.

With a score of between 60–79, there is again scope for improvement.

With a score of between 80–99, scope for improvement still exists, although it is likely to be in terms of a series of small changes and modifications rather than anything more fundamental.

With a score of 100 or more, care needs to be taken that pharmacists and staff maintain the standards being achieved and that complacency does not creep in.

- What are the obstacles to making the changes needed in order to achieve a customer-centred pharmacy, how significant are they, and how might we overcome them?

ARE THE APPARENT BENEFITS REALLY BENEFITS?

Perhaps the easiest and most useful way of identifying and assessing the benefits that customers might get from a service is to apply the 'which means that' and the 'so what?' tests; these are illustrated in Figures 3.1 and 3.2. Some pharmacies now offer home delivery of prescriptions 'which means that' patients do not have to visit the pharmacy with obvious benefits for those who are not easily mobile. The service means that they no longer have to ask friends or nursing staff to collect the prescription items for them. However, for a

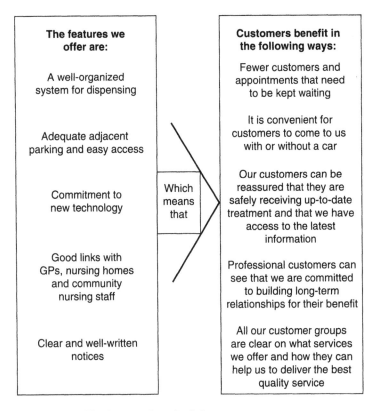

Figure 3.1:   The features–benefits link

customer who can only visit the pharmacy in the daytime the 'so what?' tests highlights that the change is of no real or direct value (although there may, of course, be the indirect benefit that because prescriptions are being spread throughout a longer day, the pharmacy will not be so crowded at peak times).

Given this, and recognizing that the benefits to customers are not always as obvious or as significant as might have been hoped or expected at first sight, Figure 3.2 can be used to identify – and, more importantly, assess – the *real* benefits of any features that you currently offer or are thinking of developing.

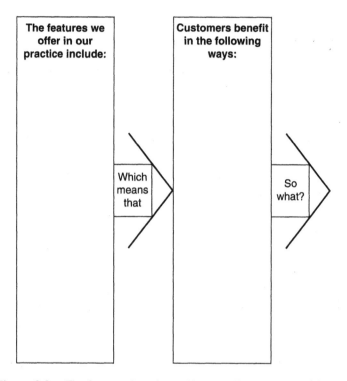

Figure 3.2:   The features, benefits and 'so what?' link

WHAT DO CUSTOMERS REALLY WANT FROM THEIR PHARMACISTS?

Before looking at the question of customer wants, it is worthwhile taking a moment to consider the real underlying needs of the customer. In most cases, needs and wants are one and the same thing, although there are instances where great care must be taken to diagnose the customer's own perception of the situation.

Whilst pharmacists might believe that their competence in dispensing might feature as one of the most important criteria for customer selection of a pharmacy, customers may take for granted accurate dispensing and want a pharmacy that also provides a good range of health care products.

MOVING AHEAD

Given the nature of these comments, the question of how the truly customer-centred pharmacy might be developed needs to be approached by considering the answer to a series of questions.

- Do we really know what levels of satisfaction and dissatisfaction currently exist amongst our customers?

- Where customers are dissatisfied, do we really know how deep and/or justified this dissatisfaction is?

- Are we really aware of the causes of customer irritation with the pharmacy and are there any common strands between any of these causes for complaint/dissatisfaction that customers might have?

- Do we really understand what leads to high(er) levels of customer satisfaction?

- Would we really be willing to make possibly radical changes in the way we operate in order to achieve higher levels of customer satisfaction?

- Have we really done enough to train our staff or do we rely upon common sense and learning from the long-established members of staff?

- How much money would we really be willing to invest in new product ranges and training facilities in order to achieve higher levels of customer satisfaction?

In the light of your answers to the various questions that we have posed in this chapter and the score that has emerged from the checklist in Box 3.2, you should have some understanding of the nature of the pharmacy's orientation and the extent to which it is really customer-centred. Our experience has shown that pharmacies can be viewed very broadly in terms of a continuum, ranging from, at one end, the inward looking and old-fashioned pharmacy in which customers know their place and dare not move from this, through to the highly customer-centred pharmacy at the other; this is illustrated in Figure 3.3.

In most cases, of course, pharmacies do not appear at one extreme or the other but are instead located at some point along the continuum. In identifying where you are on this, you should therefore

---

Box 3.3:   The customer-unfriendly business

Paddy Miles has just bought a retail pharmacy for £410 000. The turnover is £730 000 and growing at around 10% a year. However, after just a few days, the new owner is beginning to discover that there are one or two problems about which the seller kept quiet. The most immediate concerns the staff. The senior assistant, for example, sees herself to be something of a shop steward and is proving to be subtly unco-operative. Indeed, the thought that keeps going through the pharmacist's mind is that if the senior assistant was in the army, she would be guilty of dumb insolence. In addition, he feels that she is not taking on the responsibility he might reasonably expect her to. Although he has explained to her what he wants to do with the business and the role he wants her to play, he is finding it difficult to get from her the sort of commitment he thinks is needed.

Amongst the problems he has begun to identify is that she has some customers who are her firm favourites and to whom she appears to spend too much time talking. Others, however, are treated in an almost cavalier or offhand way. When faced with this and told to spend less time with her favourites, she has responded by saying, 'So you don't want me to be friendly with the customers then'.

In these circumstances, how would you go about developing a more consistently customer-friendly pharmacy?

---

focus not so much upon the specifics of the factors that characterize pharmacist-centred pharmacies and customer-centred pharmacies, but rather on the nature of the underlying picture and the extent to which this reflects the prevailing attitudes, cultures and methods of operating within your own pharmacy. Having done this, and having identified which end of the spectrum the pharmacy is currently biased towards, think about *why* the pharmacy is where it is. More often than not you will find that the nature of the pharmacy mirrors the general approach of the one or two longest serving and most senior members of the team.

SUMMARY

Within this chapter, we have focused on some of the dimensions of a customer-centred pharmacy and on how such an approach can

The pharmacist-centred pharmacy is characterized by a belief that:	The customer-centred pharmacy is characterized by:
• there is no good reason to change, because the pharmacy is among the best in the area	• a clear understanding of customers' needs and the benefits they are seeking
• apart from the occasional problem, the customer management system works perfectly	• a willingness to adapt the pharmacy, its systems and product ranges to meet customers' needs
• customers are fundamentally a nuisance	• the belief that without customers there would be no pharmacies
• the pharmacist knows what is best for the customers and what is best for the pharmacy	• an understanding of how other pharmacies (and multiples) operate and what can be learned from them
	• a listening approach
	• the development of new services
• the objective is to maximize the use of existing services	• a willingness to invest in new facilities and equipment and close services that are no longer needed
• customers know that we are here to serve them	• a willingness to deliver to customers if appropriate
• training is only effective if it relates directly to the individual's present job	• a well thought-out programme of training for all staff

Figure 3.3: The dispensing pharmacist-centred/customer-centred continuum

only be developed against the background of a clear and detailed understanding of customers' expectations. In developing a stronger customer orientation, an obvious starting point is the recognition of the distinction between features and benefits and of the need to look outside the pharmacy and evaluate what it has to offer from the customers' perspective. In the absence of this, the pharmacy will almost inevitably lack the customer focus that is increasingly being demanded and expected.

4

Environmental pressures and the parable of the boiled frog

Having read this chapter, you should:

- understand the various dimensions of the macro and micro external environments and how their patterns of interaction are capable of affecting the pharmacy

- understand the need to review the environment on a regular basis

- appreciate how the environment creates opportunities and threats

- have an insight into the ways in which the pharmacy's environment is likely to develop and become more volatile over the next few years

- understand the implications of this for approaches to the pharmacy's organization.

We commented in Chapter 2 that marketing involves a four-stage process: environmental analysis; planning; implementation; and feedback and control. Within this chapter, we focus upon the first of these and examine the significance of the pharmacy's environment, the ways in which it is changing, the implications of this and how an understanding of the probable patterns of environmental change is capable of contributing to more effective marketing planning. However, before looking at the detail of this, it is worth learning the lesson of the boiled frog.

THE PARABLE OF THE BOILED FROG

All organizations are faced with a series of environmental changes and challenges. The principal difference between the effective and the ineffective organization is how well it responds, something that was encapsulated several years ago in one of the most popular of management fables, the parable of the boiled frog. What is now referred to as 'the boiled frog syndrome' is based on the idea that if you drop a frog into a pan of hot water, it instantly leaps out. If, however, you put a frog into a pan of lukewarm water and turn the heat up very slowly, it sits there quite happily not noticing the change in its environment. The frog, of course, eventually dies. The parallels with the management and development of any organization are, or should be, obvious. Faced with sudden and dramatic environmental change, the need for a response is obvious. Faced with a much slower pace of change, the pressures to respond are far less (this is the 'we are doing reasonably well and can reassess things at some time in the future' phenomenon), with the result that the organization becomes increasingly distant from the *real* demands of its customers and other stakeholders. Given this, think seriously about whether you are one of the frogs that are sitting quite happily in a pan of increasingly hot water. If so, why, what are the possible consequences and what, if anything, are you going to do about it?

ANALYSING THE PHARMACY'S ENVIRONMENT

Although a variety of frameworks has been developed to help in the process of analysing the environment and assessing its probable effect upon an organization, the most useful of these is referred to as PEST analysis – an acronym of what are the four major dimensions of the environment for the majority of organizations: the **P**olitical/legal; **E**conomic/competitive; **S**ocio-cultural; and **T**echnological elements.

The thinking that underpins PEST analysis is straightforward and involves taking each of the four elements in turn, identifying the nature and significance of any changes that are likely to take place, in either the short or long term, and then assessing what effect these will have upon the organization. Having done this, thought can then be given to the actions and responses that are possible and/or demanded.

Although the relative importance of the four factors is likely to vary over time, and indeed their impact may be either direct or indirect, the benefits of regular environmental analysis can be considerable, and are reflected most obviously in terms of a pharmacy that is capable of behaving far more proactively, recognizing emerging opportunities and threats at a much earlier stage and taking the action that is needed to capitalize on the opportunities and minimize – or avoid altogether – the impact of any threats.

It follows from this that if you are to act in a proactive manner, you need to begin by identifying and categorizing those parts of the environment over which you are able to exert at least some small degree of control, and those which, by virtue of being totally outside your control, need to be seen as environmental constraints.

Having carried out an analysis of the environment, you can then start to develop a strategy that is far more likely to reflect the environmental pressures and realities rather than the partners' preconceived – and possibly misconceived – ideas of what is feasible.

The reality for many pharmacies is, of course, that the vast majority of external factors are constraints that can only rarely be changed or influenced to any real degree. The implications of this are, first, that the argument for monitoring the environment is inescapable since you need to shape the pharmacy so that it more accurately reflects environmental demands, and, second, that you need to structure the pharmacy so that it is sufficiently flexible to be able to respond effectively and quickly to external pressures, be they in the form of opportunities or threats.

THE STRUCTURE OF THE ENVIRONMENT

The various dimensions of the environment are illustrated in Figure 4.1. It can be seen from this that the environment is capable of being categorized not just on the basis of the PEST factors that we have already referred to, but also on the basis of their macro nature, in that they affect the nation as a whole (an obvious example would be the changing demographic patterns and, in particular, the increasing numbers of elderly people needing prescriptions and advice) and

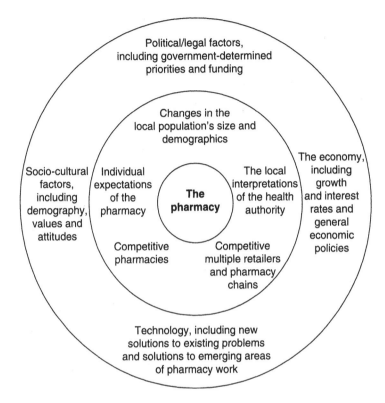

Figure 4.1:   The pharmacy environment

their micro impact, in that they have a direct and immediate impact upon the pharmacy or the local community; an example of this would be the way in which an upsurge in local levels of unemployment often has a knock-on effect upon pharmacy services in the communities affected.

Because of the ways in which the environment is the immediate or ultimate influence upon patterns of demand for the pharmacy's services, a regular environmental review is capable of providing significant insights not only into the sort of change taking place but also into the patterns of response and development within the pharmacy that are needed. Without this, it is likely that sooner or later the pharmacy will be forced into a series of reactive responses in a desperate attempt to avoid the sort of mismatch between what

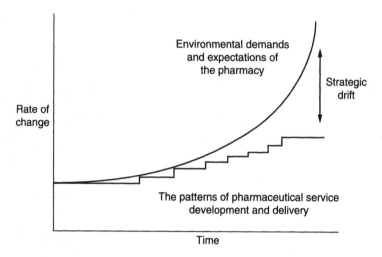

Figure 4.2: The mismatch between environmental demands and pharmacy delivery

various parts of the environment are demanding and what the pharmacy is actually offering; this mismatch is illustrated in Figure 4.2.

The phenomenon that Figure 4.2 illustrates is sometimes referred to as 'strategic drift' and is one that we have encountered in a substantial number of pharmacies that we have dealt with, and is manifested in a variety of ways. Among these are growing levels of customer dissatisfaction, a failure on the part of the pharmacist to recognize and agree how emerging opportunities might be exploited, little desire amongst the staff to carry out anything other than routine tasks, and a general weakening in the image of the pharmacy both within the community and the medical profession. Faced with this, the only response that is then possible is a radical reassessment of current environmental demands, how this is likely to change and how the pharmacy intends to respond in order to catch up.

PATTERNS OF ENVIRONMENTAL CHANGE

In looking at any environment, we can categorize it on the basis of the nature and pace of the changes taking place and the managerial/

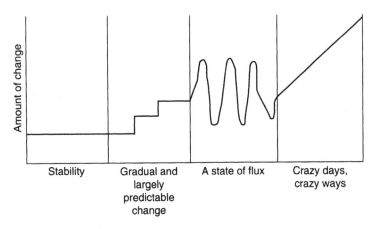

Figure 4.3: Patterns of environmental change

organizational implications of this. In Figure 4.3, we illustrate four broad patterns of environmental change: stability; gradual and largely predictable change; a state of flux; and what Tom Peters, the leading American management guru of the 1980s and 1990s, has referred to as 'crazy days'. This stage, he suggests is characterized by a large number of major, unpredictable and often seemingly malevolent environmental changes. Crazy days, he argues, call for very different patterns of management responses in which traditional approaches and mind sets are of little value. It is these new and far more innovative approaches to management that he labels 'crazy ways'.

In the case of pharmacies, the sorts of environmental change faced by pharmacies for a long time corresponded to Stage Two, that of gradual and largely predictable patterns that could be accelerated with few real problems. Over the past few years, however, it is not only the pace and scale of change that have increased dramatically, but also the degree of unpredictability. Because of this, the nature and pace of the responses that are required have escalated enormously, a recent example being the speed at which some multiple retailers have gained what was traditionally local pharmacy business. In organizational and managerial terms, the implications of this can be examined under a number of headings, particularly in terms of the need for greater organizational flexibility, better patterns of communication and far higher levels of staff training.

THE SIGNIFICANCE OF SOCIAL CHANGE

Perhaps the most significant series of changes that pharmacies will have to come to terms with over the next few years stems from the series of structural and attitudinal shifts that are taking place within society. Included within these series are:

- the growing number of elderly people and a series of other major demographic shifts

- a general increase in drug abuse and crime

- an increasing disregard for authority

- rising divorce rates

- the continual change in shopping habits in favour of supermarkets

- a greater awareness of health issues

- a greater willingness among some people to live healthier life-styles

- changing attitudes to professionals and a desire for more personal and individual treatment

- a greater willingness to complain and seek compensation

- expectations of higher service levels.

Although this is not an exhaustive list, it provides an indication of the sorts of social changes that are likely to have an impact over the next few years. Because of this, you should go through the list adding to it where necessary and assess the extent to which you feel that your pharmacy will be affected by each of the points, and then how you might respond most effectively.

Together, however, they spell out the need for more flexible and organic approaches to pharmacy organization. The alternative, a largely traditional and mechanistic structure, simply creates problems. Consider therefore, the questions that appear in Box 4.1.

In answering these, you need to give serious thought not only to the superficial changes that have been initiated in the pharmacy, but also to the rather more fundamental issues of the attitude and behaviour of everyone in the pharmacy. We know of some

Box 4.1:   How effectively has your pharmacy responded to and managed change?

1. What are the biggest changes that you feel have affected pharmacies over the past few years?

2. Which of the changes that have taken place have had the greatest effect upon your pharmacy?

3. Overall, how well do you think that these changes have been handled?

4. What have been the major problems that have been experienced in responding to and managing these changes?

5. What are the principal causes of these problems?

6. What, if anything, has been done and is being done to overcome these problems?

7. What do you see to be the major changes that the pharmacy will have to face up to over the next few years?

8. How well equipped is the pharmacy to deal with these effectively?

9. What areas of managerial strength and weakness exist in the pharmacy?

10. What messages do these areas of managerial strength and weakness send out about your ability to handle future changes effectively?

pharmacies, for example, which have installed impressive computer systems, given the exterior of the pharmacy a facelift and provided new style makeovers for the staff, but which still think and act in much the same way that they have for years with no real improvement in their organization, style of leadership or approaches to teamworking. They are now suffering the problems of poorer performance and substantially worse staff morale, aspects that led us to identify the four different types of pharmacy that are illustrated in Box 4.2.

Although there is an obvious element of parody in at least two of these profiles, there is a more serious underlying question that is concerned with the existing attitudes to change within the pharmacy,

Box 4.2:   The four types of pharmacy and their responses to change

The dinosaurs

These are the pharmacies that exist in a time warp. Life goes on as it always has, with few, if any, changes. In essence, it is the sort of pharmacy where customers can go to find the remedies their grandparents recommended. The floors are covered with linoleum and the walls are painted a shade of green that is guaranteed to induce a sense of impending doom in even the most cheerful of customers. The dispensing staff see the dispensary area as their personal fiefdom, prescriptions are an unwelcome intrusion and friendliness is seen as a sign of weakness, whilst the pharmacist regrets that weighing, pouring and counting are no longer part of the science. The competition from other pharmacies or pharmacists is generally either ignored (competition from the supermarkets is beyond the pale) or dismissed on the grounds that the shops are too bright and/or flashy. The customer base is small and declining and primarily made up of the elderly who have used the pharmacy for years and who would find the transfer to another pharmacy impossible to contemplate. Change is seen as a nuisance, a threat and largely unnecessary, with the result that the pharmacist works hard to avoid any move away from the methods that were at the cutting edge of pharmacy management in the 1920s.

The docile and contented cows that are ambling along

These are the pharmacies that have made steady if unspectacular incremental progress. The pharmacy has been spruced up, with shop fittings circa 1981, the staff have name badges, a computer has been installed for label printing and the pharmacist regularly attends pharmacist events in order to find out about the latest advances.

The sheep

This is the sort of pharmacy in which the pharmacist has latched on to and introduced every new idea that has come along in the last few years, only to replace it after a couple of months with something new. There is little evidence of planning or of a well thought-out and sustained direction for the pharmacy, but considerable evidence of a series of knee-jerk responses to a variety of half-baked ideas. The computer system is impressive. The shop displays are immediately recognizable by the glass and chrome furniture, old copies of fairly

continued

Box 4.2: *continued*

esoteric management journals in the dispensary, and the prominently displayed – and, it must be said, largely meaningless and incomprehensible – pharmacy mission statement that makes reference to breaking down barriers between customers and staff and the development of far stronger and truly meaningful interpersonal relationships taking place, even though they are quite conspicuously not working.

The pharmacist in these practices is easily identified by a wild-eyed look and messianic approach that is tempered by a growing realization that none of the numerous management innovations that have been introduced is really working in the hoped-for or promised way. Other staff in the pharmacy are recognizable by their air of weary resignation and a sense of impending doom.

The eagles

These are the pharmacies in which considerable thought has been given to the future and to the sorts of objectives that are most appropriate. These thoughts have then been reflected in a series of considered and appropriate responses that take full account of the various stakeholders' expectations. The result is a pharmacy that is well prepared to cope with the challenges of the next few years and in which complacency, staff rivalry, obstruction and self-satisfaction have no place.

The pharmacy is recognizable for its quiet efficiency as soon as you walk through the door. It is staffed by people wearing the pharmacy's uniform and a name badge, who know how to put you at your ease and genuinely seem to care. They know many regular customers by their names and make sure that the prescription system runs efficiently with no long waits for customers. The pharmacy is light and airy, has an up-to-date notice board and an ample supply of leaflets providing advice on health matters. Morale is high, the staff are motivated and, once appointed, rarely leave.

how well the pharmacy has responded to change so far, the extent to which planning for the future is going on and the quality of this planning. The question of how well the pharmacy has responded so far was touched upon in Box 4.1 and may well have highlighted issues of whether the responses to change have been planned or are largely

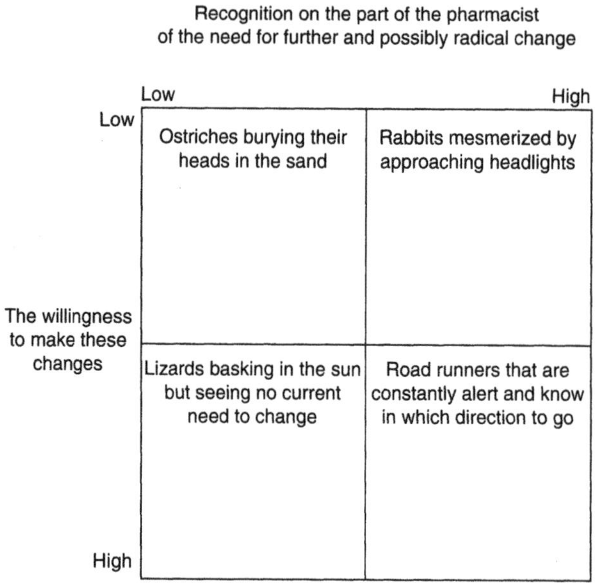

Recognition on the part of the pharmacist
of the need for further and possibly radical change

	Low	High
Low	Ostriches burying their heads in the sand	Rabbits mesmerized by approaching headlights
The willingness to make these changes	Lizards basking in the sun but seeing no current need to change	Road runners that are constantly alert and know in which direction to go
High		

Figure 4.4:   The change matrix

fortuitous. With regard to the issue of the quality of planning for the future, you need to give thought to two interrelated issues. First, the extent to which there is a fundamental recognition on the part of the pharmacists of the need to continue changing over the next few years and, second, the willingness to make these changes rather than simply responding to them. This is illustrated in Figure 4.4.

Having placed the pharmacy within this matrix, ask yourself a few straightforward questions.

- Why are we in this cell of the matrix?

- Are we happy with this? If so, what do we have to do either to stay here or improve yet further?

- If we are not happy with the current position, what are the root causes and what do we have to do to improve things?

WAYS OF IMPROVING EACH OF THE TYPES OF PHARMACY

Given the nature of the profiles in Box 4.2 and your responses to the three questions above, you need to think about how your pharmacy, be it a dinosaur or eagle, might possible develop over the next few years. In the case of the dinosaurs, there is little that will really achieve any change, short of the pharmacist retiring or being bought out. Like the dinosaurs of the past, the dinosaur pharmacies of today are destined simply to die and will reappear only in museums as a reminder of what things used to be like.

The docile and contented cows that currently are ambling along have a slightly brighter future, although just how bright this proves to be is likely to depend upon the arrival of a shining knight on horse-back (apologies for mixing the metaphors). Without the injection of some new ideas, many of which are likely to prove uncomfortable, the contented cows will continue to amble along, and will eventually illustrate radical new thinking on evolution by taking on the shape of the dinosaurs.

In many ways, the sheep represent the most interesting challenge, since the pharmacist's approach is a case study of exactly how in managerial terms you should not do things. The range of solutions here is therefore relatively small and limited either to a palace coup (look to South American politics and the guidance given by the CIA for exactly how this might be done) or an appeal to decency (the British army in the 19th century wrote the rule book on this one by giving a loaded revolver to anyone who let the side down, pointing them in the direction of a darkened room and encouraging them to do the decent thing). Either way, it comes down to what most personnel managers refer to as 'a major career change time' or 'an opportunity to pursue other interests'.

With regard to the eagles and how they might improve on what is already a pretty slick operation, there is little that can be said. Insofar as they might possibly have a problem, it is that they run the risk of achieving the very high standards they are aiming for and become complacent. However, the true eagles recognize this, guard against it and fly ever higher.

THE STEPS IN ANALYSING THE ENVIRONMENT

In Box 4.3, we provide a framework that is designed to help in the process of identifying how the environment is likely to change over the next few years, what the implication for the pharmacy are likely to be, and what the strategic imperatives are. (A strategic imperative is a 'must do' factor, in that if you fail to address it, the consequences for the pharmacy are likely to be significant.) Having done this, you can then move on to Boxes 4.5–4.8 which require you to look more specifically at the four principal dimensions of the environment that we referred to earlier (political, economic, social and technological), identify the changes taking place, assess whether these represent

---

Box 4.3:   Basic environmental beliefs, their implications and the strategic imperatives that emerge

Basic environmental beliefs

I believe that the following environmental changes will take place over the next few years:	The implications for the organization of each of these changes will be:	The strategic imperatives (the 'must-dos') that emerge from this are:
1.	1.	1.
2.	2.	2.
3.	3.	3.
4.	4.	4.
5.	5.	5.
6.	6.	6.
7.	7.	7.
8.	8.	8.
9.	9.	9.
10.	10.	10.

Box 4.4:   Bright past, bleak future?

The Village Pharmacy is a small owner-managed pharmacy with two part-time staff. The shop, which is located in a small village-like community on the edge of a town, has been losing both counter and prescription trade, and the owner is now faced with the need to decide what he is going to do.

The immediate cause of the problem is only too obvious in that a major supermarket chain has recently received a contract and has opened an in-store pharmacy just over a mile away. Looking at the figures, a gloomy picture emerges. With a gross margin of 26% on a turnover of £300 000 (down from £400 000 a year ago), staff costs of £15 000, rent and rates of £6500, £45 000 of stock, interest on the stock of around 10% (say £4500), locum costs that mean that a four week holiday costs £2400, additional overheads that are running at around 2% of turnover (say £6000), plus all the normal tax and National Insurance payments, net income this year is less than £40 000. The owner has recently been approached by the business development director of an aggressive regional chain with a take it or leave it offer to buy the business for about two-thirds of what the owner feels it is worth. Attached to the offer would be the opportunity to work for the chain as the shop manager.

In trying to decide what to do, he begins to calculate what would happen if he loses another 15% of turnover.

Faced with this, what would you recommend?

---

opportunities or threats, and what action the pharmacy needs to take.

To do this, you need to work your way through each of these areas in turn with your management team and other key members of staff, with a view to identifying, first, the nature of any changes that are likely to take place and, second, the implications of these for the pharmacy.

In doing this, use a flipchart, and brainstorm so that as many ideas as possible are generated without being evaluated or criticized. (If you are unfamiliar with the technique of brainstorming, the essence of it is that you have a short period during which as many ideas as possible are written up on to the flipchart. The main rule is that criticism is

Box 4.5: Probable PEST developments – The political/legal environment

The probable political/legal developments are …	The probable specific effects of each of these are …	Are these likely to represent an opportunity or a threat for us?	What do we need to do to capitalize upon each of the opportunities and minimize each of the threats?
•	•	•	•
	•	•	•
	•	•	•
•	•	•	•
	•	•	•
	•	•	•
•	•	•	•
	•	•	•
	•	•	•
•	•	•	•
	•	•	•
	•	•	•

forbidden at this stage so that people are not afraid to put forward their thoughts, no matter how bizarre they might seem.) Once you have done this, go back and evaluate each of the ideas before entering them in Boxes 4.5–4.8.

To help in this process of getting started, the questions that appear below might be of some help. We have deliberately posed just a few questions under each heading, with a view to you then developing the list at much greater length and in much greater detail.

Box 4.6:   Probable PEST developments – The economic/competitive environment

The probable economic/ competitive developments are …	The probable specific effects of each of these are …	Are these likely to represent an opportunity or a threat for us?	What do we need to do to capitalize upon each of the opportunities and minimize each of the threats?
•	•	•	•
	•	•	•
	•	•	•
•	•	•	•
	•	•	•
	•	•	•
•	•	•	•
	•	•	•
	•	•	•
•	•	•	•
	•	•	•
	•	•	

The political/legal framework

- What sorts of change in the current government's policies do you foresee?

- What changes do you foresee in health care priorities in general?

- What effect would a change in funding levels for the NHS have?

- What changes do you foresee in the levels of responsibility and accountability for pharmacists?

Box 4.7: Probable PEST developments — The socio-cultural environment

The probable socio-cultural developments are ...	The probable specific effects of each of these are ...	Are these likely to represent an opportunity or a threat for us?	What do we need to do to capitalize upon each of the opportunities and minimize each of the threats?
•	•	•	•
	•	•	•
	•	•	•
•	•	•	•
	•	•	•
	•	•	•
•	•	•	•
	•	•	•
	•	•	•
•	•	•	•
	•	•	•
	•	•	•

- Does the pharmacist keep up-to-date on relevant changes in the law?

The economic, competitive and provider environments

- What changes do you expect to see in economic conditions both nationally and locally?
- How will unemployment levels change locally and what are the implications for patterns of health care demand?

Box 4.8: Probable PEST developments – The technological environment

The probable technological developments are …	The probable specific effects of each of these are …	Are these likely to represent an opportunity or a threat for us?	What do we need to do to capitalize upon each of the opportunities and minimize each of the threats?
•	•	•	•
	•	•	•
	•	•	•
•	•	•	•
	•	•	•
	•	•	•
•	•	•	•
	•	•	•
	•	•	•
•	•	•	•
	•	•	•
	•	•	•

- In what ways is competition becoming more significant for pharmacies and how is this affecting you?

- What are the implications for other local pharmacies of the changes that are taking place?

- What sort of relationship do you have with adjacent pharmacies?

- What appear to be their objectives and how are they likely to develop over the next few years? Does their pattern of development have any implications for you?

- What might you learn from how other pharmacies operate?

- Is there any scope for greater co-operation? Can you pool resources? Can you refer work on a structured basis for mutual advantage?

- What changes do you expect to see in the relationships with general practices, nursing homes and other health care providers?

The social and cultural environments

- What social changes do you expect to see over the next few years?

- What are the implications for you of trends and shifts in the local population size and demographic structures?

- In what ways are customers' expectations of pharmacies changing?

- In what ways are values and life-styles changing?

- What new social and cultural pressures and priorities are emerging?

The technological environment

- How will technological changes and developments affect the pharmacy over the next few years?

- In what ways might an individual's expectations of higher technology medical solutions develop?

- What are the implications of new technological developments for the pharmacy and working methods?

- Is the management team fully up-to-date with the nature and patterns of technological developments in delivery of medical services?

- How might you use new technology to improve your range and level of services?

- Does anyone within the pharmacy have the specific responsibility for monitoring new developments and keeping the others informed?

Having gone through this exercise, you should have a far clearer and more focused view of how the pharmacy's environment is likely to

Box 4.9:   The opportunities and threats facing the pharmacy

The opportunities open to us appear to be …	Their significance (1–5) (1 = of little significance; 5 = of major significance)	The actions that are needed to capitalize upon the opportunities are …
•	•	•
•	•	•
•	•	•
•	•	•
The threats facing us appear to be …	Their significance (1–5)	The actions needed to minimize the possible impact of the threats are …
•	•	•
•	•	•
•	•	•
•	•	•

develop and what the implications of this are likely to be. Armed with this information, you should then be in a position to begin identifying in detail the sorts of opportunities and threats that currently exist, the ways in which they are most likely to develop in the near future and how they can best be handled; a framework for this appears in Box 4.9 (this framework is developed further both in Chapter 6 and, in particular, in Box 6.2 and Figure 6.2, and in Chapter 8).

SUMMARY

Within this chapter, we have focused upon the various dimensions of the environment and how an understanding of the environment, and the ways in which it is likely to change, underpins any worthwhile approach to planning. Against this background, consider the following questions.

1. Do you feel that you have a sufficiently detailed understanding of how the pharmacy's environment is likely to change over the next few years?

2. What sort of environment does it look as if you will have to face up to? (Refer back to Figure 4.3.)

3. How confident are you that you will be able to cope effectively?

4. Where do the greatest opportunities and threats appear to be?

5. Given your previous patterns of behaviour, how are you most likely to respond to any changes? Will it be largely in the form of a series of almost desperate moves, or in a much more systematic and planned manner?

6. Is there currently a mismatch between what your pharmacy is offering and what the market is really demanding? (Refer back to Figure 4.2.) If there is a gap, how significant is it and what are you doing/will you do to close it?

Finally, return for a moment to our story of the boiled frog and think not only about the lessons that emerge from this but also, in the light of your responses to the questions that we have raised within this chapter, what sort of frog you really are.

5

Planning for success (part one): assessing your planning skills

> Having read this chapter, you should:
>
> - understand more clearly what you want from planning
> - have a greater understanding of the planning skills and abilities possessed by you and your colleagues.

SO WHAT DO YOU WANT FROM PLANNING?

It has long been recognized that planning is generally a relatively easy and straightforward exercise and that the development of a truly worthwhile plan takes only a little more time and effort than that involved in preparing one that is mediocre. The problems that many organizations face come therefore not at the planning stage but are instead related to the ways in which the plan is implemented. Far too often, for example, too few resources are put into the process of implementation and responsibilities are only loosely allocated, with the result that objectives are not achieved within the hoped-for timescales. Faced with this, the all-too-common reaction, particularly when the environment is changing rapidly, is to see planning as being of little real value and the process as little more than a hollow exercise.

If, however, the processes of planning and implementation are seen to be interconnected, responsibilities are properly allocated and someone within the pharmacy takes on the task of 'driving' the plan, the benefits can be considerable and reflected in a far tighter focus and much higher levels of motivation and performance.

However, for many managers – and we include pharmacists within this – planning runs the risk of taking on what is sometimes loosely referred to as 'motherhood' status. In other words, it is warm, reassuring and difficult to argue against. Before we go any further, therefore, you need to consider seven simple questions:

1.   Why are you bothering to plan?

2.   What will the plan be used for?

3.   How will it be used?

4.   Who will be involved in the planning process?

5.   ·Who will write it (and how)?

6.   Who will manage and drive it?

7.   What measures of success will you use?

THE TWO APPROACHES TO PLANNING

In working with a wide variety of organizations over the years, it has become apparent that, when it comes to planning, there are two broad approaches. The first is characterized by an emphasis on producing a lengthy, detailed, highly polished and professional-looking plan which is then, either literally or figuratively, filed until the start of the next year's planning cycle.

The second approach, and the one to which we want to give emphasis in this chapter, gives full recognition to the benefits of the planning process in that it provides a forum for a detailed review of the environment, objectives, priorities, resources, strengths and weaknesses, and to the alternative patterns of proactive development that exist. This is then reflected in the plan itself, which represents a *working document* in that it is used on a daily/weekly basis to manage the pharmacy. Given this, the answer to the first of the seven questions posed above has to be that any plan that is developed must be realistic and designed to make a major contribution to the management of the pharmacy, rather than to satisfy any guidelines or expectations of a bank. (A rule of thumb that we often use as a first step when talking to pharmacists or other professionals about their planning process simply involves looking at the pharmacy's planning document. If it is dog-eared, has been annotated and is relatively slim, the chances are that it is used on a day-to-day basis as a working document. Presented with a fat and pristine plan, we can almost guarantee that the plan is not really used and that we will be able to sell the pharmacy some consultancy advice on how to improve their planning – and implementation – processes.)

It follows from this, therefore, that you need to think seriously about developing a planning culture within the pharmacy in which the process of planning is taken seriously rather than being only a once-a-year ritual.

BEING REALISTIC ABOUT YOUR PLANNING SKILLS

Perhaps one of the most common complaints that we hear from professionals on a regular basis is that they qualified in order to practise their particular discipline rather than to become professional managers. Although we have a certain sympathy for this view, few pharmacists today are able to duck their management and planning responsibilities.

However, recognizing that pharmacists currently vary enormously in terms of their planning abilities, a first stage in developing an effective planning process involves being realistic (perhaps brutally honest would be a better phrase) about the planning skills of each of the partners within the pharmacy. To do this, begin with the matrix that appears in Figure 5.1, which requires you to categorize individuals

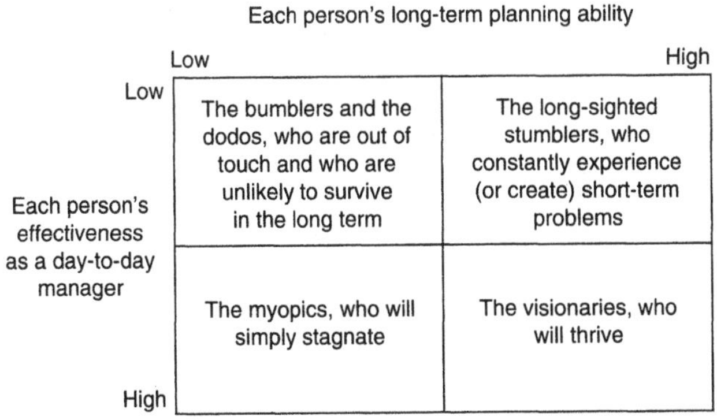

Each person's long-term planning ability

	Low	High
Low	The bumblers and the dodos, who are out of touch and who are unlikely to survive in the long term	The long-sighted stumblers, who constantly experience (or create) short-term problems
High	The myopics, who will simply stagnate	The visionaries, who will thrive

Each person's effectiveness as a day-to-day manager

Figure 5.1:   The short- and long-term management skills matrix

The ability of each person to manage

	Low	High
Low	The incompetent meddlers	The opt-outs and the ostriches
High	The danger pharmacist	The super pharmacist

Their willingness to manage

Figure 5.2: The four management styles

on the basis of two dimensions: their apparent long-term planning abilities and their skills in day-to-day management. Using this matrix, identify where your pharmacy is located. The picture that emerges from this should give you a reasonable insight into the overall quality of management and the planning strengths that exist within the pharmacy, whether there is a need to strengthen these, and who might be best equipped to take on the initial responsibility for planning. In completing this matrix, you are also arriving at a measure of what is loosely referred to as organizational capability; that is, the pharmacy's capacity for handling change and moving ahead in the right direction.

Against this background, you should then move to Figure 5.2, which enables you to categorize yourself on the basis of your *willingness* to manage and your *ability* to manage; the four types that this produces are discussed in Box 5.1.

SUMMARY

Within this chapter, we have quite deliberately tried to adopt a reasonably light-hearted tone in order to drive home an important message and, in the case of Box 5.1, would say again that we have identified uncanny parallels between pharmacists and GPs. Given the far greater emphasis upon, and indeed the need for, planning in the current climate, it is essential that before going any further you have a clear understanding of the managerial and planning strengths that exist within the pharmacy. Without this understanding, there is a danger that you will start with the assumption that all partners have an equal ability and that the responsibilities for both planning and

Box 5.1:   The four types of pharmacist-manager

In the light of a study that we conducted amongst managers of medical practices in 1993 to find out how they viewed their GPs as managers, we identified four types of pharmacist-manager: the superpharmacists, the dangerpharmacists, the opt-outs and ostriches, and the incompetent meddlers. Subsequently, in our work with lawyers, we have found that this categorization can be applied with unnerving ease. We therefore leave it to you as a pharmacist to work out which most nearly describes your own style.

The **superpharmacist** proved to be an all too rare – and un-nerving – species, immediately recognizable by an evangelical gleam in his or her eye, an almost pathological commitment to change, a passion for computerization, and a love of plans, planning and staff information notes. Superpharmacists tend to put enormous emphasis on mission statements for the pharmacy, partners' away days in order to decide on the future objectives and the shape of the pharmacy, staff motivation, and scrupulous record keeping. Their briefcases bulge with business plans and a mobile phone sits next to the counter.

The **dangerpharmacists** are the pharmacists, who, despite few obvious managerial skills, are intent on demonstrating to staff throughout the firm that they are in charge and are full of ideas (few of which are original and fewer still of which are understood). They tend to use management jargon indiscriminately and are intent on bringing about change; in managerial terms they are the equivalent of someone practising as a pharmacist having failed their Boy Scouts or Girl Guides first aid badge. All too often, the changes they make and the systems they introduce are either inappropriate or, because of a lack of planning and commitment, fail to achieve the hoped-for results. Despite this, they insist on being involved in everything and often feel that their staff have no real skills or abilities. Because of this, they have an almost neurotic compulsion to give orders to anyone and everyone. Like the superpharmacists, dangerpharmacists can be recognized in a number of ways, most obviously by the trail of confusion and/or destruction they leave behind and their insistence upon being consulted about every aspect of the pharmacy. Insofar as they have a pet phrase, it is likely to be either 'Didn't I tell you about that? I suppose I must have forgotten', or 'Why has it gone wrong? Can't anyone around here do anything right?'

continued

Box 5.1:   *continued*

Those in the third category – the **opt-outs and ostriches** – are something of a disappointment in that although they have a well-developed ability to manage, they either do not see themselves as managers, and consequently leave others to do it, or still have not come to terms with the way in which pharmacy has changed over the past few years. Tolerant of a degree of chaos, they often develop delegation to a fine art. Insofar as they can be recognized by what they say – as opposed to what they do not do – it is likely to be something along the lines of, 'I didn't come into pharmacy to be a manager, I just want to get on with being a pharmacist'.

The fourth category – the **incompetent meddlers** – proved to be surprisingly common and a source of enormous frustration. These are the pharmacists who consistently fail to complete vital records on time, rarely if ever tell the staff what is going on or where they are going, see no need to plan, frequently change their mind for no apparent reason, insist on being ·consulted (a bit like danger pharmacists), and either wouldn't recognize a business plan if it landed on their desk or would not be able to find it amongst the mess of free gifts from reps, unanswered telephone message, half-eaten sandwiches and still-to-be-read articles from the medical press.

Box 5.2:   Refocusing the business

Keith Lewis is a bright young pharmacist who worked for a major national pharmacy chain for two years before working with an independent for 12 months. He has managed to get financial backing and has found a proprietor who is on the verge of retiring and who is willing to sell the business. The proprietor has invested relatively little in the business over the past 15 years and there is, as the proprietor readily admits, the need for 'a bit of money to be spent'. The site appears to offer considerable potential, particularly as a group of GPs is shortly to move their practice from their current premises ¾ mile away to a new purpose built building just 250 metres along the road. The pharmacist perceives this to be an opportunity to become part of the primary health care team and wants to develop the professional service side of the business with screening, information leaflets and so on.

What advice would you give to make sure that the full potential is realized?

implementation can be shared equally. If our experiences with numerous managers in a wide variety of organizational types over the past 20 years are at all typical, this is simply not the case, It is the recognition of this and the picture that emerges from the various matrices used in this chapter that leads us to suggest that it is only after you have identified the level and nature of the planning and managerial skills within the pharmacy, that the question of who is to be responsible for developing, and then subsequently implementing, the plan can really be decided.

In summary, therefore, consider the following questions.

1. What overall picture emerges from the various matrices?

2. Does it appear that you have sufficient long-term planning skills amongst the partners and management? If not, what are the probable consequences of this and what might you do to overcome the problem?

6

Planning for success (part two): developing the marketing plan

Having read this chapter, you should:

- understand the nature, purpose and benefits of planning

- have an appreciation of the sorts of problem that are typically encountered in planning

- understand the structure of the marketing plan and the inputs that it requires

- be aware of how the assumptions that underpin the plan subsequently act as 'drivers' of the plan

- appreciate how stakeholders' needs can and should be taken into account

- have an understanding of the sorts of factors that affect the effectiveness of the plan's implementation.

Against the background of our comments in Chapter 5 and, hopefully, a better understanding of the planning skills and abilities that exist within the pharmacy, we can now turn our attention to the question of how best to prepare an effective marketing plan.

THE THREE DIMENSIONS OF PLANNING

We commented in Chapter 5 that plans often fail because too little attention is paid to issues of implementation. Equally, they fail because the objectives that have been set are either too ambitious or fail to reflect the realities of the environment and/or the organization's strengths and capabilities. Recognizing this, planning, which is designed to provide the organization with a sense of direction and purpose, must take place against the background of a clear and detailed under-standing of three principal factors:

1.   the nature and demands of the environment

2.   the objectives and expectations of the pharmacist and staff

3.   the pharmacy's strengths, weaknesses and overall levels of capability.

THE STRUCTURE OF THE MARKETING PLAN

Although there is no one model of the ideal marketing plan, it is relat-ively easy to identify the 12 areas that need to be included within any worthwhile and useable planning document. These are illustrated in Box 6.1 and then brought together diagrammatically in Figure 6.1.

DEVELOPING AN EFFECTIVE PLAN

Planning is based on asking – and answering – three principal questions.

1.   Where are we currently?

2.   Where do we want to go?

3.   How are we going to get there?

The significance of the first of these – where are we currently? – has been highlighted by the ex-chairman of ICI and star of BBC television's *Troubleshooters* series, Sir John Harvey-Jones:

'There is no point in deciding where your business is going until you have actually decided with great clarity where you are now. Like practically everything in business, however, this is easier said than done.'

This stage of the planning process is therefore concerned very largely with identifying the pharmacy's real strengths and weaknesses, along

---

Box 6.1:   The elements of the marketing plan

1. The summary or overview

2. The situational analysis that includes:

    *   the assumptions that have been made about environmental pressures and demands, and the assessment of the opportunities and threats that currently exist and which seem likely to emerge during the period covered by the plan
    *   the assessment of the pharmacy's strengths and weaknesses, its overall level of capability and the identification of any significant gaps

3. The implications of the analysis of strengths, weaknesses, opportunities and threats

4. The principal assumptions underlying the plan

5. The statement of the mission and the short- and long-term marketing objectives

6. The statement of the strategy that is to be pursued

7. The detail of the tactical actions needed

8. The allocation of responsibilities and timescales

9. The resource implications of the plan

10. Feedback mechanisms

11. The performance measures that are to be used to assess ongoing performance

12. The procedures for review and control

---

with the nature of any opportunities and threats that currently exist or which seem likely to emerge during the period that is to be covered by the plan. Having done this, you can then move on to the question of the direction in which you want to take the pharmacy, something that involves not only the development of a clear statement of objectives but also a vision of the sort of pharmacy that you are trying to develop. Against this background, you can then turn your attention to identifying how this vision and the objectives might best be obtained.

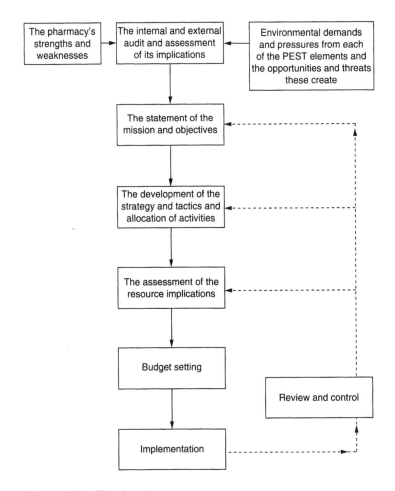

Figure 6.1:   The planning process

STEP ONE

Where are we currently?

How to conduct a SWOT analysis that is really worthwhile
SWOT analysis (Strengths, Weaknesses, Opportunities and Threats) has proved to be one of the most commonly used – and abused – managerial and planning tools of the past decade. There are several reasons for this, the most obvious perhaps being that the technique's

apparent simplicity has lulled its users into a false sense of security with the result that all too often the outcome of the analysis is far too bland and meaningless to provide a worthwhile base for planning. Given this, how then can SWOT analysis be made more rigorous and meaningful? The guidelines that emerge from having experienced these sorts of problem with a variety of different types of organization are straightforward:

- Concentrate upon building a picture of the pharmacy as a whole by carrying out a series of preliminary analyses that focus upon different parts of the pharmacy such as prescribing and counter sales. By doing this, you are not only far less likely to miss some of the detail that needs to come from a SWOT, but you will also gain a far greater insight into how different parts of the pharmacy are operating and how they need to develop.

- Do not conduct the analysis on your own, but instead use it as an opportunity for getting the pharmacy staff to pool ideas.

- Always look at strengths and weaknesses from the viewpoint of the customer and other stakeholders. In this way, you avoid making a series of warm, reassuring and bland motherhood statements about the pharmacy and can concentrate upon identifying how it is really seen from the outside.

- In looking at strengths and weaknesses, start with a broadly unstructured approach in order to get ideas flowing, but gradually pull the points together under a series of headings so that you can build up a picture of the pharmacy's different dimensions. The sorts of headings that you might use in doing this include:

    - the pharmacists and locum pharmacists
    - the skill levels of the pharmacy assistants
    - the pharmacy premises, including their location
    - the administrative procedures
    - the information technology that is being used
    - financial issues and any investment needs
    - relationships with customers
    - relationships with GPs, community nursing staff and the health authority
    - relationships with suppliers
    - the general and specific reputation of the pharmacy.

- In looking at the external environment, concentrate upon those parts of the environment that are likely to have a direct rather than an indirect effect upon the pharmacy.

- Avoid the temptation simply to list strengths, weaknesses, opportunities and threats, since this tends to lead to what we can refer to as a 'balance sheet' mentality in which you take comfort from the way in which, for example, the number of strengths identified outweighs the number of weaknesses. Instead, spend the time evaluating each of the points identified and then rank them in order of importance; a framework for doing this appears in Box 6.2.

Box 6.2: Identifying the pharmacy's strengths, weaknesses, opportunities and threats

Strengths	Significance
Weaknesses	Significance
Opportunities	Significance
Threats	Significance

- Concentrate upon identifying how the results of the analysis can be used. In the case of strengths, for example, there has to be a matching opportunity; without this, the strength is of little real immediate value. Equally, in the case of weaknesses, think about how each weakness can be overcome or its significance reduced. In the case of threats, again think about how their impact can be neutralized or reduced, and possibly turned into an opportunity; the framework for this appears in Figure 6.2.

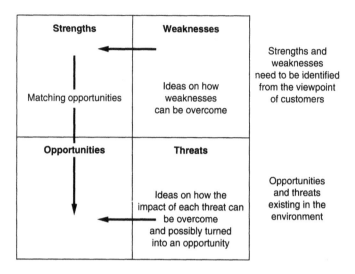

Figure 6.2:   The customer-oriented SWOT

DEVELOPING A VISION AND A MISSION FOR THE PHARMACY

A considerable amount of management research has in recent years highlighted the importance of vision and mission statements and the role that they are capable of playing in providing staff with a sense of direction and purpose; in the case of pharmacies, the overall statement of vision would be concerned with a general expression of the sort of pharmacy that you are trying to create in the medium to long term. An obvious example of this would be that of a pharmacy that has the strongest reputation locally for the quality of customer care and up-to-date services and facilities. (The position of the vision within the planning hierarchy is illustrated in Figure 6.3.) Such a pharmacy might have a vision statement along the lines of 'To be a high quality pharmacy providing services to the community within a radius of [10] miles of [Anytown], with a particular emphasis on continuous improvement in standards whilst also achieving maximum profitability'.

You might therefore ask yourself the following question:

- To what extent is there currently a *shared* and *explicit* vision amongst the staff of the sort of pharmacy we are trying to develop?

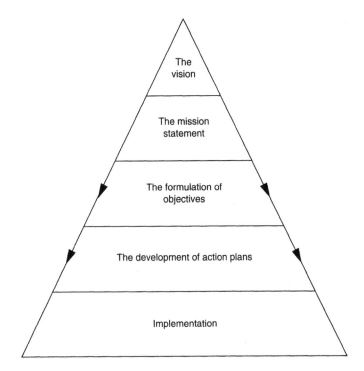

Figure 6.3: The planning hierarchy

In the majority of pharmacies that we have come across, there appears to have been relatively little detailed thought or discussion of this sort of issue, with the pharmacists having concentrated instead upon a whole series of shorter term issues. It is, however a funda-mental part of the planning process, since it represents a collective statement of what in the long term you are really trying to achieve.

The significance of a shared vision needs therefore to be seen in terms of the broad framework that it is capable of providing and the influence that this should then have upon both the subsequent mission statement and the sorts of objectives that are set.

Given this, think again about the question that we posed earlier ('To what extent is there a shared and explicit vision?') and consider raising it at the next management meeting, with a view to getting an explicit statement of the sort of pharmacy that, between you, you are trying to create. To help with this, you might usefully also consider the three questions below.

1. What do we want the pharmacy to be like and known for in, say, five years time? (In answering this, think about the range of products and services offered, the reputation and size of the pharmacy, its location and desired level of profitability.)

2. How realistic is this vision?

3. What do we need to do if we are to translate this vision into reality?

Against this background, you can then move on to the development of the mission statement. A mission statement represents a statement of core values and is again part of the framework within which plans are prepared. It is for this reason that at least one commentator has referred to the mission as 'an invisible hand' that guides staff to work in particular ways. There are numerous examples of good mission statements in retailing, two of which are illustrated in Box 6.3. (We have quite deliberately chosen these not from pharmacies, but from businesses with which you will be familiar on a more general basis.)

Having looked at many hundreds of mission statements over the past few years – some of which have been good, some bad, and others simply a tribute to the ability of managers to fantasize – there are several lessons that emerge which are worth keeping in mind when developing a mission statement for your pharmacy. They include:

•   make sure that it gives a general direction and encompasses key values; it should not include goals or actions

•   keep it short, otherwise staff will probably never read it, let alone remember it or really understand it

•   make sure that it focuses upon fundamental issues and reflects core pharmacy values that will neither need changing nor be changed every six months or so

•   make sure that it is believable and not made up of a series of unrealistic 'wish' statements

•   make sure that it is exciting and inspirational

•   make sure that it is communicated and explained to staff throughout the pharmacy and that a copy is posted in a prominent position in the waiting room

Box 6.3: Mission statements

Sainsbury has stated its mission as being:

- To discharge the responsibility as leaders in our trade by acting with complete integrity, by carrying out our work to the highest standards, and by contributing to the public good and to the quality of life in the community.

- To provide unrivalled value to our customers in the quality of the goods we sell, in the competitiveness of our prices and in the choice we offer.

- In our stores, to achieve the highest standards of cleanliness and hygiene, efficiency of operation, convenience and customer service, and thereby create as attractive and friendly a shopping environment as possible.

- To offer our staff outstanding opportunities in terms of personal career development and in remuneration relative to other companies in the same market, practising always a concern for the welfare of every individual.

- To generate sufficient profit to finance continual improvement and growth of the business whilst providing our shareholders with an excellent return on their investment.

Marks & Spencer's mission is broadly similar:

- To offer our customers a selective range of high quality, well designed and attractive merchandise at reasonable prices.

- To encourage our suppliers to use the most modern and efficient techniques of production and quality control dictated by the latest discoveries in science and technology.

- With the co-operation of our suppliers, to ensure the highest standards of quality control.

- To plan the expansion of our stores for the better display of a widening range of goods (and) for the convenience of our customers.

- To simplify operating procedures so that our business is carried on in the most efficient manner.

- To foster good human relations with customers, suppliers and staff.

- recognize that although a first draft can be prepared by one person, the creation of one that is truly worthwhile can only be done as the result of a detailed discussion of values and aspirations.

Putting these guidelines into practice involves focusing upon two interrelated dimensions: the **customer-related issues** (what customers' needs do we intend meeting and how?); and **key values** (what central or core values, such as quality and levels of customer service, and which we are simply not prepared to compromise on, will it encompass?). Both of these are encompassed in a mission statement we came across recently:

> 'As a pharmacy, our mission is to provide our customers with the highest levels of care at all times by understanding, anticipating and responding to their full range of needs, providing a highly accessible service that is of the highest quality.'

This statement incorporates a number of the guidelines that we highlighted earlier and whilst scope exists for some improvement, it has so far proved to be of enormous value within the pharmacy in question, in that it has highlighted the values that are seen to be at the heart of that pharmacy.

Against the background of these comments, consider the following questions:

- Does your pharmacy currently have a mission statement? If so, does it reflect the sorts of guideline that we referred to earlier and incorporate the values that really are at the heart of the pharmacy, or is it simply empty rhetoric?

- If the pharmacy does not yet have a mission statement, what value do you think might be gained from developing one?

STEP TWO

Where do we want to go?

How to set worthwhile objectives

To be effective, a planning system must be goal driven. The setting of clear and meaningful objectives is therefore a key step in the

Box 6.4:   The ten guidelines for worthwhile objectives

Objectives need to be:

1. Hierarchical, going from the most important to the least important

2. Quantifiable, so that performance against target can be measured at a later stage

3. Limited in number. If you set a large number of objectives, it is likely that you will not only lose sight of at least some of them, but also make the process of developing a strategy that is capable of achieving all of them unnecessarily difficult. You should therefore concentrate on identifying the most important areas in which objectives need to be set, and then use these as the basis for developing the strategy

4. Realistic and a true reflection of the pharmacy's strengths, the environmental opportunities, your contractual obligations and the level of the capability, rather than being a series of wishful thoughts

5. Consistent, rather than mutually incompatible

6. Related to well-defined time periods

7. Stated explicitly with no scope for ambiguity

8. Based upon the pharmacy's strengths and designed to help overcome weaknesses

9. Communicated to staff throughout the pharmacy, with the implications for how they operate being explained to them

10. A reflection of the various elements of your mission statement.

marketing planning process, since unless it is carried out effectively, everything that follows will lack focus and cohesion. The purpose of setting objectives is therefore to provide the pharmacy with a sense of direction. In addition, however, they can be used as a basis for motivation as well as a benchmark against which performance and effectiveness can subsequently be measured.

The ten guidelines for setting worthwhile and meaningful objectives are straightforward and illustrated in Box 6.4.

Against the background of these guidelines, consider the following questions:

- What are the pharmacy's current short term and long term objectives?

- To what extent do the pharmacy's objectives conform to the ten guidelines above?

- How often are the objectives reviewed in detail?

- How often and in what detail is performance against objectives measured?

- How much detailed thought is given to the process of developing and implementing the actions needed to achieve these objectives?

IDENTIFYING THE AREAS THAT YOUR OBJECTIVES SHOULD COVER

In setting objectives for the pharmacy, you need to aim for a balance between several areas including:

- the pharmacists' expectations

- regulatory constraints

- the expectations and needs of staff

- the issues associated with the long-term development of the pharmacy, its premises and equipment

- customers' expectations of the quality and levels of service they will receive.

Although this is not an exhaustive list, it provides a useful framework for identifying the sorts of objective that you might need to consider developing. Taking each of these in turn, you should therefore list the key points that need to be considered. In the case of customers, for example, you might identify issues such as how quickly they expect to be served, how easy it is to see the pharmacist, how long they might have to wait for a prescription if the drug is not in stock, how long it takes to deal with telephone calls and so on.

Having identified the key issues under each of these and any other headings that you see to be important, you can then begin the process of refining the list of objectives, making them more specific and attaching timescales, so that some will be essentially short term ('all reception staff to have reached a pre-determined level of information technology capability within 12 months'), whilst others, such as the complete refurbishment of the pharmacy's premises, will be longer term.

Having done this, you are then in a position to begin reviewing the objectives with a view to seeing which, if any, are unrealistic either in terms of their magnitude (in other words, they are simply too ambitious) or that are unlikely to be achieved in the short term but can be achieved over a slightly longer period. In doing this, you are trying to identify the nature and significance of any gaps that exist between your expectations and the ability of you and the staff throughout the pharmacy to meet these expectations. With this information, you can then either modify the objective or increase the degree of attention and the resources devoted to its achievement.

As an example of gap analysis, consider the objective of increasing the profit by 50% over the next three years. By giving detailed thought to what is likely to be involved in achieving this, it may become apparent that it can be achieved only by recruiting more staff, opening new services, making substantial changes to administrative procedures, and the development of a more aggressive retailing culture.

Having considered these implications, you may then decide that whilst the objective is laudable, the pharmacy is simply not willing to make the changes that would be needed for it to be achieved. If this is the case, you need to go back and either modify the objective by watering it down or crossing it out altogether. It may, of course, be at this stage that significant differences of opinion emerge as to the future of the pharmacy. You may feel, for example, that you have developed a shared vision of the future but the realization of what is actually needed to put it into effect may highlight fundamental differences of opinion. This is one of the benefits of a rigorous planning process, since it is far better to realize that such differences exist before embarking upon implementation. You must then either modify your vision and mission statement or even decide (hopefully amicably at this stage) to go separate ways. If such fundamental differences do exist, it is pointless to ignore them and early remedial action is always the best option to pursue.

STEP THREE

How are we going to get there?

Developing the action plans that will work

Having identified your short- and long-term objectives, you should be in a position to begin developing action plans. In doing this, you often need to be very specific and to pay considerable attention not only to the question of what needs to be done, but also to who is to be responsible for each element and what intermediate measures or checks of performance are needed; a framework for this appears in Box 6.5.

Once you have done this, you need to recognize that implementation is often the most difficult part of the planning process, since it is all too easy to be side-tracked by the sheer pressure of day-to-day activities. In the light of this, give thought to three questions:

1. Who within the pharmacy is to be responsible for driving the plan?

2. How often do you intend holding review meetings to check on the progress being made and whether any corrective action is needed?

3. What sort of feedback are you going to give the staff on how well or bad the plan's implementation is proving to be?

The question of who is to drive the plan is important, since whoever takes on the responsibility for this has to recognize from the outset that much of the plan's subsequent success will depend upon how well the job is done. It is therefore essential that in deciding who is to do this, that:

-   they are fully committed to the plan and understand each of its elements in detail

-   they have the authority and enthusiasm to make sure that no-one loses sight of what the plan involves and what their contribution to its implementation should be.

Box 6.5: The action planning framework

Objectives	Actions needed to achieve these objectives	Allocation of responsibilities	Intermediate performance measures
Short term			
•			
•			
•			
•			
•			
•			
Long term			
•			
•			
•			
•			
•			
•			

HOW LONG SHOULD THE PLAN BE?

Perhaps the most frequently asked question that we have been faced with in discussing marketing plans with professional practices concerns the plan's length. Our advice is always the same: keep the plan as straightforward, short and simple as possible and, above all, make sure that it is capable of being used as a *working document*. Second, having written it, do not make the mistake of filing it or assuming that its implementation will take place as if by magic. The answer to the question of length is therefore a little difficult, in that it is impossible to say whether it should be ten pages or 20. Instead, we would remind you again of the benefits of the planning process (assuming, of course, that is has been done properly), in that it forces you to look not only at the detail of the pharmacy's strengths and weaknesses, but also at the environment and the objectives that you intend pursuing. We would also highlight the way in which planning can clarify a considerable number of issues by bringing them into sharper focus and again, assuming that it has been done properly, lead to better patterns of communication, understanding and commitment throughout the pharmacy. Having said all of this, the answer to the question of length has to be that it is not particularly important, but that the two overriding characteristics of worthwhile plans are, first, that they are used as working documents and reflect a planning culture in which full recognition is given to the benefits of the various stages of the analysis and so on, and second, that they help you to achieve objectives that are seen to be worthwhile within the pharmacy.

THE NINE PLANNING PITFALLS TO AVOID

In working with a variety of pharmacies and helping the pharmacists to develop marketing plans, we have encountered a number of common planning difficulties that, once you are aware of them, are relatively easy to overcome. They are:

1. a tendency to assume that budgeting and planning are one and the same thing; they are not

2. the development of too many and unrealistically ambitious objectives

3. an unclear vision of the sort of pharmacy that the partners are trying to develop

4. an emphasis upon analysis rather than decisions and implementation

5. poor internal communications with the result that levels of staff understanding and commitment to the plan are less than they should be

6. seeing planning as a ritual rather than an activity capable of making a real contribution to the development of the pharmacy

7. inadequate resourcing and poor implementation procedures

8. failing to allocate responsibilities sufficiently

9. poor monitoring, feedback and control.

Against the background of our comments so far, it should be apparent that there is a set of simple guidelines for effective planning. These include the need to:

- treat the plan as a working document (do not file it)

- make it realistic and based on the pharmacy's real strengths and weaknesses

- keep it simple and user friendly

- make sure that it reflects opportunities and comes to terms with any threats that exist or seem likely to emerge

- ensure that it reflects a long-term vision of the sort of pharmacy you are trying to create

- make sure that it improves teamworking and commitment

- see it as an opportunity to question the conventional wisdom

- allocate responsibilities clearly

- make sure the timescales are realistic

- monitor performance and do not be afraid to take corrective action where it is needed

- emphasize communication by getting others involved from the outset – osmosis is only rarely a useful or adequate method of communication

- make sure that the plan can be and is implemented.

SUMMARY

Within this chapter we have focused upon the three principal steps of the planning process. Insofar as it is possible to identify the element that characterizes effective planning, it would have to be the involvement and commitment of all staff to both the development and the implementation of the plan. Without this, any attempt at planning is likely to prove to be of little real value. Recognizing this, there are three final guidelines that you need to bear in mind.

1. Avoid the ivory tower syndrome in which the senior partner develops the plan in isolation, presents it to other partners and staff, and then expects a full-blooded commitment to its implementation.

2. Make sure that staff throughout the pharmacy are involved in the process from as early a stage as possible and are then made fully aware of the contribution that is expected of them in its implementation.

3. Always provide feedback on how well or how badly the pharmacy is performing, highlighting what the next stage of development will be.

7

Using the marketing audit and the marketing effectiveness review to assess the true level of the pharmacy's capability: revisiting your strengths and weaknesses

Having read this chapter, you should:

- understand the nature and role of the marketing audit

- be aware of the audit's components

- understand how to conduct a marketing audit.

One of the biggest and most common problems faced by organizations, regardless of their type or size, is that plans all too often fail to come to fruition. There are several explanations for this, the most common being that the objectives set are too ambitious, too little thought is given to the activities needed to achieve the plan, and, faced with day-to-day pressures, staff lose sight of what they are trying to achieve. Because of this, and as we pointed out in Chapter 6, effective marketing planning must be based upon a clear statement of *realistic* objectives and a detailed understanding of what the pharmacy is really *capable* of achieving. Although there are several ways in which the pharmacy's capability can be measured, one of the most useful and straightforward tools for this is the *marketing audit*, which requires you to focus upon a series of dimensions, such as the pharmacy's strategy, its systems, the levels of productivity, and so on, with a view to identifying the real detail of the pharmacy's strengths and weaknesses. The audit can then be taken a step further by conducting a review of marketing effectiveness (a framework for this appears in Box 7.2).

Although the idea of looking at the pharmacy's strengths, weaknesses, opportunities and threats was raised in Chapters 4 and 6, our experience has shown that professionals often produce better and more tightly focused SWOT analyses if they are faced with a framework of questions, rather than having to generate them themselves. It is this which, therefore, represents the real rationale for this chapter.

THE COMPONENTS OF THE AUDIT

The marketing audit involves looking in detail at six areas:

1. *The environment:* how are environmental forces currently developing and how are they likely to change in both the short and long term?

2. *The pharmacy's strategy:* how well formulated are the objectives and the strategy, and how well suited are they to the current and future environments?

3. *The organization:* how capable is the pharmacy of implementing any action plans that are developed?

4. *The systems:* how appropriate and effective are the pharmacy's systems for planning and control?

5. *Productivity:* how cost-effective are the different areas of the pharmacy?

6. *Facilities and resources:* how well suited are the pharmacy's facilities to what you are trying to achieve?

Quite deliberately, the audit we discuss here is not all embracing, but is instead designed to encourage you to think about specific aspects of the pharmacy. Supplementary questions can therefore be added to make it more directly relevant to an individual pharmacy. In working your way through the six sections, you should therefore continually pose two fundamental questions:

- What are the implications of my answer for the pharmacy?

- What are we/am I going to do about these implications?

For the results of the audit to be worthwhile, a few simple rules need to be kept in mind:

1. The process must be comprehensive and cover all parts of the pharmacy rather than just a few known trouble spots.

2. It must be systematic and follow an orderly sequence of steps.

3. It must be independent and not influenced by personal feelings, relationships or pre-conceived notions.

WHO SHOULD CONDUCT THE AUDIT?

With regard to who should conduct the audit, there are several possibilities. The first of these, which is also the cheapest and often the fastest, involves the pharmacist taking on the responsibility. There are, however, potential disadvantages in this, in that, with the best will in the world, he or she may not necessarily be totally objective. Because of this, within a number of the pharmacies that we have dealt with, we have established a small task force consisting of the pharmacist, one of the pharmacy technicians, and one or two pharmacy assistants. By doing this, awkward questions are more likely to be addressed and a generally broader perspective brought to the exercise.

As you complete each section of the audit, you need to assess the implications of your answers with a view then to identifying the sorts of action and response that these demand of the pharmacy; the framework for this is illustrated in Box 7.1. As an example of this, if the strategy audit suggests that the pharmacy's objectives are either not clearly stated nor sufficiently well communicated to the staff throughout the pharmacy, the steps to correct this need to be spelled out, responsibilities allocated and acted upon and a reporting back date agreed. Equally, if the productivity audit suggests that certain areas have cost levels that are too high, an action plan to deal with this again needs to be developed.

Having completed all six sections of the audit and conducted the marketing effectiveness review, the findings can then be pulled together in the form of the sort of SWOT (Strengths, Weaknesses, Opportunities and Threats) framework that we discussed initially in Chapter 4 and then in greater detail in Chapter 6, with thought being

Box 7.1:   The findings and implications of the marketing audit

Findings	Implications	Actions required
The environmental audit • • • •		
The strategy audit • • • •		
The organizational audit • • • •		
The systems audit • • • •		
The productivity audit • • • •		
The facilities and resources audit • • • •		

given to the actions needed to exploit strengths, convert any weaknesses to strengths and threats to possible opportunities (see Figure 6.2).

THE MARKETING AUDIT

The environmental audit

- What effect will forecasted trends in the size, age distribution and regional distribution of the population have on the pharmacy?
- What changes in attitude towards pharmacies are taking place amongst the public?
- What changes are taking place in consumers' life-styles and values that will have a bearing on our customer groups?
- How do our current customers perceive and rate the pharmacy?
- In what ways are our customers' expectations changing?
- What new services are likely to be required over the next few years?
- To what extent are our customers' current expectations being met?
- How might customers best be categorized (e.g. young/old, coming for prescriptions or purchasing other items)? What are the expected rates of growth of each of these categories?
- How are other pharmacies nearby perceived?
- How do other pharmacies operate and what might we learn from them?
- How do different groups of customers appear to make their choice of pharmacy?
- How are the expectations of stakeholders likely to change over the next few years?

The strategy audit

- Are the pharmacy's short-term and long-term objectives sufficiently clearly stated?

- Are they understood by everyone in the pharmacy?

- Is there generally agreement on their validity?

- Do the objectives provide sufficient guidance for planning and control purposes?

- Are the objectives appropriate given the demands of customers and the external environment?

- Is there a well-formulated overall strategy?

- If so, are staff aware of the strategy and the nature of the contribution that they are expected to make to it?

- Have sufficient resources been made available for the objectives to be achieved?

- Have the resources been optimally allocated across the various customer groups?

- Are there any new services or product ranges that we might offer?

- Are there any existing services that we might offer to new customer groups?

- Are there any services that might benefit from minor or major changes being made to them?

- Are there any services or product ranges that we currently offer that should be dropped?

- Is there any scope for offering more of our existing services to our existing customers?

- What are the pharmacy's promotional objectives?

The organizational audit

- Is there someone who has direct responsibility for planning and monitoring performance? If so, does this person have adequate authority?

- Are responsibilities within the pharmacy clearly spelled out and understood?

- Are the lines of communication and working relations between staff operating as effectively as they might?

- Are lines of authority within the pharmacy clearly spelled out?

- Is there any scope for more delegation of routine tasks to support staff?

- Are there any individuals within the pharmacy who need more training, motivation, supervision or evaluation?

- Have staff undergone all the relevant training?

- Do staff appraisals take place regularly? Is there evidence that they are effective?

- Is there sufficient teamworking?

- What conflicts exist within the pharmacy?

- Do you hold regular brainstorming sessions in order to identify how levels of customer service might be improved?

- Is the task of motivation taken sufficiently seriously, or is it assumed that all staff will always be well motivated?

- Are briefing and feedback sessions held on a regular basis?

- Is an open managerial style in operation?

The systems audit

- Is the system for identifying the significant happenings outside the pharmacy working effectively?

- Is the planning system well conceived and effective?

- Are realistic targets set for staff?

- Is there an adequate monitoring system in place so that performance is measured objectively?

- Are control procedures (monthly and quarterly) to ensure that the annual plan objectives are met operating effectively?

- Is sufficient provision made to monitor, analyse and evaluate the costs of various services?

- Is the pharmacy organized to ensure that new ideas are generated and evaluated?

- What mechanisms exist to ensure that levels of customer satisfaction are being monitored?

- Is there a complaints procedure in place and are complaints regularly reviewed to detect trends and take appropriate action?

- Are the computer systems working effectively and are they adequate for the ways in which the pharmacy will probably develop?

The productivity audit

- What formal mechanisms exist to ensure that all cost areas are reviewed on a regular basis?

- Do any activities appear to have excessive costs?

- What steps are being taken to:

  – control costs
  – reduce costs?

- Are brainstorming sessions held on a regular basis in order to identify how levels of productivity might possibly be improved and how stock mark downs might be reduced?

- Do there appear to be any unnecessary procedures or processes within the pharmacy?

- Are there any procedures or processes that might usefully be modified?

The facilities and resources audit

- How do customers view your premises?

- What changes do you need to make to improve them?

- Is the pharmacy adequately resourced to achieve the objectives that have been set?

- Are the displays attractive and 'customer friendly'?

- In which areas is further investment needed?

- What obstacles do customers experience in visiting the pharmacy?

Having conducted the audit, there are several questions that need to be considered:

- What picture of the pharmacy emerges?
- What areas within the pharmacy do you need to pay attention to in both the short and long term?
- What courses of action do you need to take?
- Who is to be given the responsibility for each of these?
- What are the resource implications of any changes that are needed?

One further question that needs to be raised concerns the issue of cause and effect. Where something has gone wrong, or levels of performance are not as high as they might or should be, you need to spend time identifying *why* this has happened and *who* is primarily responsible. In doing this, the purpose is not to point the finger of blame but is instead designed to highlight the nature of any training that might be needed to overcome a skills problem and/or whether a change in the allocation of responsibilities might be appropriate.

The audit findings can then be taken a step further by conducting a review of marketing effectiveness; the framework for this appears in Box 7.2.

The review involves focusing in turn, upon five areas:

1. the customer philosophy
2. the marketing organization
3. marketing information
4. the strategic perspective
5. operational efficiency.

By working through each of these, an overall measure of effectiveness can be arrived at, this then being extended by looking at each of the five sections with a view to identifying the area(s) in which the pharmacy appears particularly weak.

Box 7.2:   The marketing effectiveness review

Customer philosophy   Score

1.   To what extent do you recognize the need to
     organize the pharmacy to satisfy specific customer
     and market demands?

   - The pharmacy philosophy is to sell existing and
     new services and products to whoever will buy them.   0
   - The pharmacy attempts to serve a wide range of
     markets and needs with equal effectiveness.   1
   - Having identified market needs, the pharmacy focuses
     upon specific target markets in order to maximize
     the pharmacy's growth and potential.   2

2.   To what extent is the marketing programme tailored to
     the needs of different market segments?

   - Not at all.   0
   - To some extent.   1
   - To a very high degree.   2

3.   Does the pharmacy adopt a systems approach to planning,
     with recognition given to the interrelationships between
     the environment, suppliers, customers and competitors?

   - Not at all, the pharmacy focuses solely upon its
     existing customer base.   0
   - To some extent, in that the majority of its effort goes
     into serving its immediate and existing customer base.   1
   - Yes. The pharmacy recognizes the various dimensions
     of the marketing environment and attempts to reflect
     this in the pharmacy's marketing programme by taking
     account of the threats and opportunities created
     by change within the system.   2

Marketing organization

4.   To what extent does the pharmacist attempt to control
     and integrate the marketing effort?

   - Not at all. No real attempt is made to integrate or
     control the various dimensions of the marketing
     programme, with the result that it is disorganized
     and lacks focus.   0

continued

Box 7.2: *continued* Score

- To a limited degree, although the levels of control and co-ordination are generally unsatisfactory. 1
- To a very high degree with the result that the marketing effort works well. 2

5. What sort of relationship exists between the staff?

- Generally poor, with frequent complains that unrealistic demands are made. 0
- Generally satisfactory, although the feeling exists that each individual works to serve his or her own needs. 1
- Overall very good, with individuals working together well in the interests of the pharmacy as a whole. 2

6. How well organized is the process for the development of new services?

- Not very well at all. 0
- New services are developed but in a spasmodic way. 1
- New services are well researched, quickly developed and achieve good results. 2

Marketing information

7. How frequently does the pharmacy gather information about its customers and competitors?

- Seldom, if ever. 0
- Occasionally. 1
- Regularly and in a highly structured way. 2

8. To what extent is the pharmacy aware of the potential and profitability of different market segments, customers and the various products and services offered?

- Not at all. 0
- To some degree. 1
- Very well. 2

9. What effort is made to measure the profitability of different services and product lines and the effectiveness of any marketing expenditure?

- None at all. 0
- Some, but not in a regular or structured way. 1
- A great deal. 2

continued

Box 7.2:   *continued*   Score

The strategic perspective

10.   How formalized is the marketing planning process?

- The pharmacy does virtually no formal marketing
  planning.   0
- An annual marketing plan is developed.   I
- The pharmacy develops a detailed annual
  marketing plan and a long-range plan that is
  updated annually.   2

11.   What is the quality of thinking that underlies the current
marketing strategy?

- The current strategy is unclear.   0
- The current strategy is clear and is largely a
  continuation of earlier strategy.   I
- The current strategy is clear, well argued and well
  developed.   2

12.   To what extent does the pharmacy engage in contingency
thinking and planning?

- Not at all.   0
- There is some contingency thinking but this is not
  incorporated into a formal planning process.   I
- A serious attempt is made to identify the most
  important contingencies and contingency plans are
  then developed.   2

Operational efficiency

13.   How well is the pharmacy's thinking on marketing
communicated and implemented down the line?

- Very badly.   0
- Reasonably well.   I
- Extremely successfully.   2

14.   Do the partners do an effective marketing job with the
resources available?

- No. The resource base is inadequate for the objectives
  that have been set.   0
- To a limited extent. The resources available are
  adequate but are only rarely applied in an optimal
  manner.   I

continued

Box 7.2: *continued*   Score

- Yes. The resources available are adequate and
  managed efficiently.   2

15. Does the pharmacy respond quickly and effectively to
    unexpected developments in the market-place?

    - No. Market information is typically out of date and the
      pharmacy's responses are slow.   0
    - To a limited extent. Market information is reasonably
      up-to-date, although the pharmacy's response
      times vary.   1
    - Yes. Highly efficient information systems exist and the
      pharmacy responds quickly and effectively.   2

The scoring process
Each pharmacist works his way through the 15 questions in order
to arrive at a score. The scores are then aggregated and averaged.
The overall measure of marketing effectiveness can then be assessed
against the following scale:

0–5	=	None
6–10	=	Poor
11–15	=	Fair
16–20	=	Good
21–25	=	Very good
26–30	=	Superior

With a score of 10 or less major questions can be asked about the
pharmacy's ability to survive in anything more than the short term,
and any serious competitive challenge is likely to create significant
problems. Fundamental changes are needed, both in the pharmacy's
philosophy and the organizational structure. For many pharmacists in
this position, however, these changes are unlikely to be brought about
by the existing management, since it is this group which has led to the
current situation. The solution may therefore lie in major changes to the
management of the pharmacy.

With a score of between 11 and 15 there is again a major
opportunity to improve the pharmacy's management philosophy and
organizational structure.

With a score of between 16 and 25 scope for improvement exists,
although this is likely to be in terms of a series of small changes and
modifications rather than anything more fundamental.

With a score of between 26 and 30, care needs to be taken to
ensure that the proactive stance is maintained and that complacency
does not begin to emerge.

Source: Adapted from Kotler P (1991) *Marketing Management: analysis,
planning, implementation and control.* Prentice Hall, Englewood Cliffs, NJ.

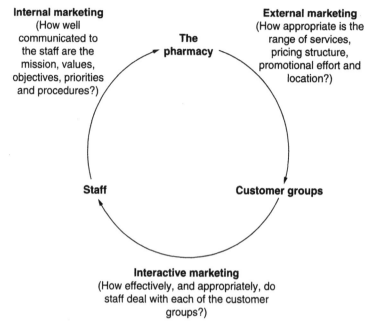

Figure 7.1:   External, internal and interactive marketing

SUMMARY

By completing the marketing audit and then the review of the marketing effectiveness, you should have a far deeper understanding of the pharmacy's marketing capabilities. This deeper understanding can then be applied to Figure 7.1, which is designed as a simple framework to highlight those areas in need of attention.

Beginning with the interface between the pharmacy and its customers, consider the nature of the external marketing effort and, in particular, the appropriateness of the pharmacy's range of services, the levels of expertise, issues of quality, the pricing policy, the promotional effort and the location of the offices. Turn then to the interface between the pharmacy and its staff and consider the nature and effectiveness of the internal marketing processes. How well communicated, for example, are the pharmacy's objectives and priorities? Finally, turn to the staff–customer interface and consider how well, or badly, this operates.

Taking these points together, what do they tell you about the pharmacy and its areas of strength and weakness?

8

Developing the pharmacy's marketing mix

Having read this chapter, you should:

* understand the various elements that make up the marketing mix

* have an appreciation of the nature and significance of the role played by the mix within the marketing process and of the ways in which managing the mix is capable of affecting the demand for the pharmacy's services.

We first made reference to the marketing mix in Chapter 2, suggesting that it consists of seven dimensions – the product/service, promotion, place, price, people, process management and physical elements. Together, these elements, which are sometimes referred to as the 7Ps, make up the marketing tool kit that is used to shape the profile of the pharmacy that is presented to the world.

Within this chapter, we focus upon each of the seven elements in turn and then, against this background, discuss how they can be brought together in the form of a coherent marketing programme and action plan.

THE 'HARD' AND 'SOFT' ELEMENTS OF THE MIX

Although we typically refer to the mix in terms of the 7Ps, it is possible to divide the mix into two distinct parts – the **'hard'** elements and the **'soft'** elements. The hard elements consist of the product/service; the price; the forms of promotion; and the price/ location in which the service is delivered. The soft elements then consist of the people who deliver the service (the pharmacist, pharmacy technician and assistants); the form of process manage- ment (how customers are dealt with from the very first to the very last form of contact); and the physical evidence (what does the pharmacy look like and what image does it convey?).

Because many customers use pharmacy services frequently, they typically assume that, until proved wrong, the quality of the products and the advice offered is high. They therefore tend to arrive at their perceptions of quality and value largely on the basis of the soft factors, such as the pharmacy staff, the pharmacy premises, the retail displays and so on. It is for this reason that particular care needs to be given to these areas in marketing pharmacy services.

THE PRODUCT/SERVICE

Almost invariably, the starting point for any discussion of the marketing mix has to be the product or service offered, since it is this that provides the basis for virtually all other marketing decisions. In the case of pharmacies, the 'product' that customers receive is, of course, the products available and the advice given (see Figure 8.1) and is made up of three distinct dimensions: the service's attributes, its benefits and the nature of the support services. These are illus- trated in Figure 8.1.

- The **service attributes** are associated with the core pharmacy service itself and are made up of the various procedures.

- The **service benefits** are the various elements that customers perceive as meeting their needs – this is sometimes referred to as the 'bundle of satisfactions'. Included within this is the perceived and actual effectiveness of the advice given or products supplied and the reassurances that the customer is given.

- The **support services** consist of all the elements that the phar- macist provides in addition to the core service. These would typically include the pharmacy assistants and their manner, how the telephones are answered and correspondence dealt with, and the relationships that exist between the pharmacist and the various

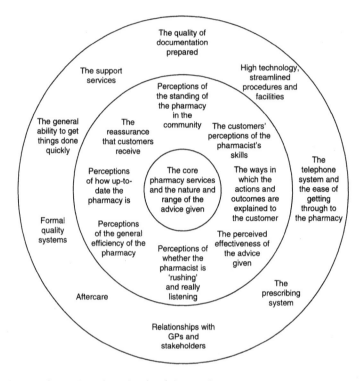

Figure 8.1: The three levels of the product or service

customers and other stakeholders, such as the local GPs, nursing home managers and district nurses.

In looking at Figure 8.1, there are several issues that emerge that are of potentially considerable significance. The first of these is the extent to which the support services are capable of setting the tone for any customer visit. Following on from this, is the way in which benefits are capable of being influenced not so much by reality, but by the customer's perceptions; it might be useful at this stage to refer again briefly to our discussion in Chapter 3 of what customers really want from their pharmacies. The third factor is that, against this background, competence in giving advice about drugs and other treatments, and the quality and efficacy of the products are often taken for granted by customers and, in a customer-centred pharmacy in particular, are the areas which they are least likely to question.

Given the nature of these comments, you might usefully consider the questions that appear in Box 8.1.

Box 8.1: Checking out your support services

The support services

- Is the pharmacy's phone system capable of handling the volume of calls you receive, or do customers often find themselves listening to an engaged tone?
- Are *all* staff sufficiently approachable, courteous, helpful and knowledgeable?
- Is the prescriptions system accurate?
- Has it been designed for the convenience of customers, or for staff?
- Are the stock record systems as good as they might be in the light of the recent advances in information and communications technology?
- Is there a general culture within the pharmacy of getting things right first time and on time?
- Are the pharmacy's relationships with other professionals as satisfactory and well developed as they might be?
- What scope exists for changes and improvements *for the customer* in each of these areas?

Service benefits: the bundle of satisfactions

- Do you have a detailed understanding of how customers perceive the pharmacy?
- How do customers appear to perceive the pharmacy in each of the following areas:
  - the advice given
  - the level of pricing
  - the general efficiency of the pharmacy
  - how up-to-date the pharmacy is
  - how quickly it gets on with the job?
- In what areas does there appear to be scope for improvement? What would be involved in making these improvements, and what obstacles would be encountered?

continued

Box 8.1:   *continued*

The core service

- What range of products and services do you currently offer?
- What scope exists for developing the profitability of each of these product ranges and services?
- What scope exists for extending these services?
- Are there any services currently offered that, for one reason or another, you should consider dropping?

In answering this final set of questions, there are two models – the product life cycle and the Ansoff matrix – which are commonly used in marketing and which might be of help in structuring your thinking; these are illustrated in Figures 8.2 and 8.3.

The product life cycle is, in many ways, one of the best known and straightforward of marketing models. It is based on the idea that any product or service has a finite life and that during this life there is a need to manage it in particular ways, depending upon the position it has reached.

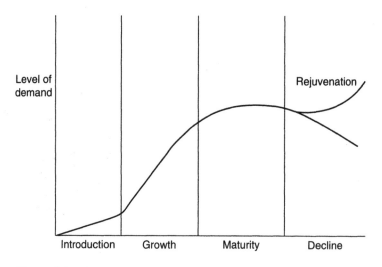

Figure 8.2:   The product life cycle

The majority of the products and services offered by pharmacists are, by their very nature, likely to be in the mature phase. However, if the pharmacist is to develop over the next few years and exploit the opportunities either that currently exist or which offer scope for development, there is a need to consider what additional services might be introduced or, in the case of some of the services currently offered, might be encouraged to grow.

To use the life cycle as a planning tool, you need therefore to begin by positioning each of your products/services on the curve in Figure 8.2. Having done this, take each of the services in turn and ask whether scope exists for its expansion and growth. If it does, think about the sorts of action that would be needed for this and what degree of growth might be possible. Considerable opportunities for development undoubtedly exist in many pharmacies, although in order to realize this potential, a series of possibly significant investment steps and skills development would be needed.

Where the demand for services appears to have stopped growing and has reached maturity, several possibilities exist. The first involves managing the service in such a way that it stays almost indefinitely in profitable maturity by ensuring, for example, that the amount of advice given remains constant and that levels of efficiency in this area are improved. An alternative approach would involve the decision to expand the pharmacy by opening a new service or merging with another pharmacy. Above all, of course, you need to guard against the gradual decline of the pharmacy, in either absolute or relative terms, as the result of a series of external changes such as increased competition from supermarkets or a change in policy by a local surgery.

Having used the product life cycle as the first step, you need then to think about how the Ansoff matrix can contribute to planning. The matrix, which is illustrated in Figure 8.3, involves initially looking at your existing services and markets with a view to identifying the scope that exists for:

1. extending existing products/services into new or untapped market sectors (e.g. home delivery for housebound patients)

2. developing new products/services for existing markets (e.g. introducing new services and promoting them to your existing customers)

3. developing new products/services for new or untapped markets (e.g. products and services for people with a disability).

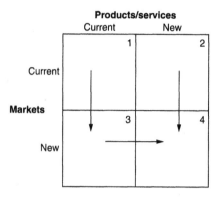

Figure 8.3: The Ansoff matrix

To use the matrix, begin by listing in the top left hand cell of the matrix as many of your existing services as you can. Having done this, use brainstorming to generate as many ideas as possible about how all or some of these might be moved into Cell Two. Try then to identify a range of new services that might be developed and offered to your existing markets (Cell Three) and, in turn, how these might be extended into Cell Four.

Box 8.2:   Creating your own future: developing stronger links with manufacturers rather than the NHS

Situated in a small market town, Drugs-U-Like is a large pharmacy with a well-developed NHS and counter trade business and an annual turnover of just over £1 million. Over the past two years, the owner has seen a gradual decline in the local shop base as the community has undergone a number of changes. Looking at the future, she realizes there are relatively few opportunities to increase the dispensing income, since the needs of the two local surgeries are already being met. Because of this, she has started to look at the opportunities for working more closely with some of the manufacturers and drug companies that have an interest in developing new health care markets, particularly disease state management. As a first step, they have started looking at the potential of asthma care.

How would you go about the process of identifying and assessing the potential of this sort of development?

Having generated these ideas, the next step involves assessing their viability by giving detailed thought to what would be involved in developing each service and market, whether this would prove to be cost-effective, and indeed whether this would be a development that, individually, the partners would welcome. In doing this, there is a further framework that can be of help; this is illustrated in Box 8.3 and Figure 8.4. To use the matrix in Figure 8.4, you need to begin by using the first column of the table in Box 8.3 to list as many areas of customer need as possible. Having done this, complete the second column which is concerned with the pharmacy's ability and willingness to service effectively each of these areas of customer need.

Box 8.3:   Customer needs and the pharmacy's ability to service these needs

Areas of customer need	Ability of the pharmacy to service each area of customer need
•	High/Low*
•	High/Low*
•	High/Low*
•	High/Low*
•	High/Low*
•	High/Low*
•	High/Low*
•	High/Low*

*delete as applicable

The next stage involves positioning each of these areas in the appropriate cells of the matrix in Figure 8.4. From the picture that emerges, you should then be in a position to identify those areas in which you might usefully concentrate some of the pharmacy's future energies and those from which you might possibly either withdraw, or at least reduce your focus. In the case of the money makers, for example, there is an obvious incentive to increase the pharmacist's effort. With those that fall into the areas for consideration, detailed

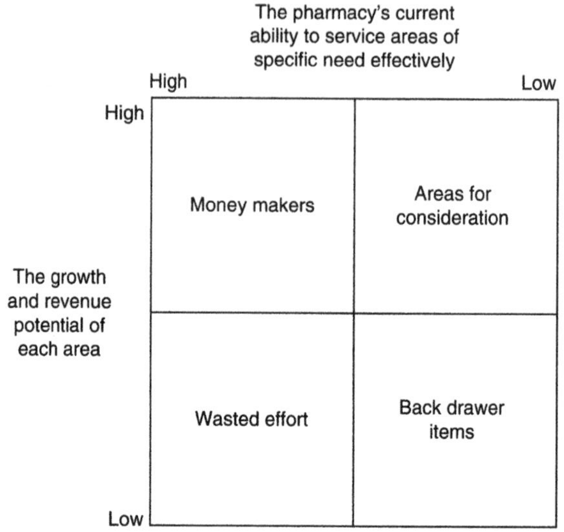

The pharmacy's current
ability to service areas of
specific need effectively

High   Low

	High	
High	Money makers	Areas for consideration
The growth and revenue potential of each area		
	Wasted effort	Back drawer items
Low		

Figure 8.4:   Customer needs and the pharmacy's match matrix

thought needs to be given to the various ways in which the pharmacist's efforts might possibly be channelled in these directions; the obvious area, of course, from which at least some of this resource might come is the wasted effort cell. Equally, serious thought needs to be given to the future of those activities that appear in the back drawer cell.

PROMOTION

Were pharmacies allowed to advertise themselves directly, there are several ways in which this could be done. However, before discussing some of the ways in which this might be done, you need to give thought to the image that you would like to create for the pharmacy. Is it, for example, that of a highly innovative, thrusting, dynamic and high technology pharmacy or one that is wedded to more traditional values? The answer to this will depend in part on the pharmacist and the premises, and in part on the types of customers you deal with. In some instances, for example, customers might well be disconcerted by what they see to be an overly modern and aggressive approach in what has traditionally been a very conservative pharmacy.

In thinking about how you will manage this part of the marketing mix, you should therefore begin by considering four questions:

1. What sort of image does the pharmacy currently have?

2. What sort of image do you, as the pharmacist, want to create?

3. What sort of image do your customers want and what will they feel most comfortable with?

4. What sort of image do other local pharmacies have?

Having done this, think about the wide variety of ways in which customers build up an image of the pharmacy. Typically this includes the age and manner of the pharmacists, the type and location of the premises, the ways in which the telephone is answered, the age and appearance of the pharmacy staff, the premises, the state of the equipment, point of sale material and the notices displayed, letters and letter headings, word of mouth and so on.

Recognition of this should give you a better understanding of the number of areas to which you will have to pay attention if you do decide to make any real change to the image that currently exists. In some cases, of course, some of the areas that we have identified can be changed at relatively low cost; the pharmacy windows and point of sale displays, leaflets and the letter headings are obvious examples. In other cases, however, changes will either be far more difficult, time-consuming and expensive, or simply not open to modification; the age and manner of the pharmacist and staff tend to spring to mind as the most obvious examples of the sorts of constraint which you would have to work around.

It should be apparent from these comments that there is probably very little that can be gained from playing around with just one or two promotional elements, and that a far more focused effort is likely to be needed. Box 8.4 should help in achieving this.

Against the background of your answers to these questions, spend some time thinking about the complete spectrum of factors that contribute to the pharmacy's image; in addition to those that we identified at an earlier stage in this section, there may be:

•   publicity in local newspapers

Box 8.4:   The promotion check-up checklist

- What overall image does the pharmacy currently have?

- What image do you want to create?

- How big a shift is going to be required in order to achieve this?

- In what ways might each of the promotional elements contribute to this new image?

- How big is the promotional budget for the next 12 months?

- Who will have the specific responsibility for developing and implementing the new image?

- What design skills do you have within the pharmacy? (Never forget that highly developed design skills are relatively rare and that you will probably save a lot of time and effort by going to a design shop from the outset rather than trying to do it yourself or letting one of the pharmacy assistants do it 'because she's creative').

- the pharmacy's leaflets and brochures

- the notices in the pharmacy

- the entry in Yellow Pages and other directories

- letters to customers, suppliers and other stakeholders (not just the letter heads and style of the letter, but also the type of paper and envelopes).

In each case, try to be objective by standing to one side and asking yourself what you would think of each of these if you were looking at them for the first time. Having done this, consider how each one might be improved. (Never be afraid to look at what other pharmacists and other professionals such as doctors, accountants, surveyors and so on are doing, with a view to learning from them.) Also try a brainstorming session. For example, what scope exists for:

- using the records system to target certain groups of customers with a personal letter to tell them about a particularly relevant service?

- running a question and answer column in the local newspaper or a trivia quiz at Christmas?

Having gone through this exercise, concentrate on developing the action plan that will help to achieve and reinforce the image that you are trying to create. In doing this, never lose sight of three golden rules:

- Have a clear 'house style' that is used on all forms of promotion.

- Keep messages simple.

- Always emphasize the benefits that customers will receive.

With these in mind, you can then move on to the sort of action plan that appears in Box 8.5.

Box 8.5:   **The promotion action plan**

The image that we want to create is that of a pharmacy which is:

The ways in which we will do this will include:

	Key messages	Timing	Responsibility
• The pharmacy's leaflets and brochures			
• Yellow Pages and other directories			
• Publicity in local newspapers			
• Letters to the customers			
• Notices in the pharmacy			
• The pharmacy's newsletter			
• What staff tell customers			
• The layout and decor of the waiting areas			

PLACE AND THE PHYSICAL ELEMENTS

For our purposes here, the place and physical elements of the pharmacy's marketing mix can be discussed in tandem, since they are concerned with three interrelated factors:

1. the location of the pharmacy

2. its accessibility

3. its general ambience and the messages that customers receive from it, both internally and externally.

In evaluating this part of the mix, you should therefore give consideration to several questions.

1. How conveniently is it located? (Although in the short term you might not be able to change the location, there is almost certain to be scope in the longer term.)

2. Are there opportunities to set up new branches?

3. How accessible is the pharmacist?

4. How often does the prescription system run late (and how many customers are affected)?

5. What does the design, layout and cleanliness say about the pharmacy?

6. Are there sufficient distractions for customers while they are waiting? Examples would include notices, topical and up-to-date magazines but no clock (if you are running late there is no point in providing a constant reminder for the customer).

7. How does it compare with the premises of other health care professionals?

8. Would you feel comfortable waiting for prescriptions?

PRICE

In any discussion of the pharmacy's marketing mix, price often proves to be the most difficult to come to terms with. For some customers and products, price is relatively unimportant particularly if it means the treatment relieves pain. However, whilst price is important for the majority of customers, it is not necessarily the cheapest pharmacies that will attract the most customers. Customers typically seek value for money and if additional benefits are offered and perceived, then premium prices on certain products are more likely to be paid. In looking at the price element of the mix, it is therefore perhaps easier to focus on issues of cost and, in particular, on just how cost-effective each element of the pharmacy really is. Given this, think about the following questions:

- How detailed is our understanding of the costs of each major dimension of the pharmacy?

- Are there any areas in which costs are unnecessarily high?

- In what ways and in what areas might we be more cost-effective?

- What scope exists for adding value to the services offered?

PEOPLE

In our earlier discussion of the product/service component of the mix, we highlighted the significance of customer perception and how this is influenced by the manner, behaviour and responses not only of the pharmacists, but also of the other staff. Because of this, the effective management of the people element of the mix has to be seen as a crucial part of the pharmacy's marketing effort, since it is capable of making or breaking the marketing programme. Consider therefore, the following.

Pharmacy staff

- How rigorous is your selection procedure for staff?
- What initial and subsequent training do they receive?

- Are staff encouraged to work in teams and do these teams work effectively?

- Do you encourage or demand a certain standard of dress? Do you have a uniform that staff are required to wear?

- What effort has gone into customer care training?

- What problems do you appear to have amongst your staff?

- What are working relationships like?

- Are there sufficient support staff of the right sort and with the right skills to enable you to achieve the pharmacy's objectives?

The pharmacist and pharmacist locums

- Are the pharmacists and locums fully up-to-date with medical and administrative procedures?

- Have they been properly trained in how to handle customers effectively, or do they just rely upon common sense? (Never forget that common sense is an all too rare commodity.)

- What additional training will they require over the next few years?

- Are working relationships between the pharmacists satisfactory?

- Are the working relationships between the pharmacists and the other pharmacy staff as effective as they might be?

Looking at the pharmacist overall:

- do you have the right blend of skills and experience for what is being demanded of pharmacists in the mid to late 1990s?

- what are levels of motivation and morale like?

In the light of your answers to these questions, you should be in a better position to begin the process of identifying in greater detail the skill and knowledge gaps that exist and which are likely to affect the customer's experience and hence their perceptions of the pharmacist.

PROCESS MANAGEMENT

The final part of the mix is concerned with the ways in which customers and information are handled. Although we have already made a number of references to issues such as how customers are handled both by the staff and the pharmacist, it is worth posing just a few more questions. How, for example, are customers addressed? Is it in a relatively formal way or as 'Luv', 'Duck' or, as we heard on one memorable occasion, 'Mate'? How are customers addressed by the pharmacists and staff when handing over prescriptions? Whatever approach is used, think clearly about how you would feel if you were the customer in these circumstances.

The second dimension of process management is concerned with the ways in which the various systems within the pharmacy operate, including the customers' records systems, filing systems and the accuracy of the relevant recording process. The questions that you should therefore consider under this heading include:

- are we making as much use of information technology as we might or should?

- how might the various systems be developed?

- what information do we need to make the pharmacy work more effectively and deliver a higher level of customer service?

- do we have a clear idea of how we might do this?

DEVELOPING THE ACTION PLAN

Having looked at each of the individual elements of the marketing mix, you need to begin the process of pulling them together in the form of an action plan; a framework to help with this appears in Box 8.6. To complete the framework, start by identifying your objectives under each of the six headings. (Remember that, although we refer to the 7Ps of the marketing mix, for the purposes of our discussion here we have amalgamated the place and physical elements.) Then move on to list, in as much detail as possible, the action steps that will need to be taken in order to achieve the objectives.

However, recognizing that not every objective or action is of equal importance or equally pressing, try then to assess the degree of priority and the timescales over which the various courses of action should take place. From here, move on to identify the broad levels of cost that will be incurred and then, finally, begin the process of allocating responsibilities.

	Objectives	Summary of the actions needed to achieve the objectives	Degree of priority	Time scales	Costs	Responsi- bilities
Box 8.6:	The marketing mix action planning framework					
Product or service						
Promotion						
Place/ physical elements						
Price						
People						
Process management						

FOCUSING THE MARKETING EFFORT

As in life generally, so it is that in marketing it is only rarely possible to be all things to all people. Because of this, any marketing programme for the pharmacy needs to reflect the needs and expectations of each of the different types of customer that you are currently dealing with or intend focusing your marketing effort upon in the future. There are various ways in which existing and prospective customers can be categorized. In marketing terms this categorization is referred to as market segmentation, targeting and positioning (see Figure 8.5).

The thinking behind what is sometimes labelled STP marketing is straightforward and can be expressed most readily in terms of the fact that because the needs, wants and expectations of customers differ – sometimes significantly – any worthwhile marketing pro-gramme needs to be based upon a recognition of these differences, which are then reflected either in the nature of the product/service that is offered and/or in the way in which it is offered.

In terms of *how* this might be done, begin by using Figure 8.5 to develop a picture of the market and the most meaningful bases for market segmentation. Having done this, identify those segments which you feel offer the greatest potential for your pharmacy. To do this, you need to think about the extent to which the pharmacy's capabilities and specialisms match the needs and expectations of each of the segments that have been identified. The third step involves deciding upon the positioning strategy that you intend adopting in each of the segments. (Positioning, in these circum-stances, relates to your general strategic and competitive stance and, in particular, to the question of the services and values for which you want the pharmacy to be known.)

Given the nature of these comments, consider the following questions:

- In what ways might current and prospective customers be most effectively segmented?

- How do the needs, wants and expectations of each of these seg-ments differ?

- To what extent do the pharmacy's capabilities match the needs and expectations of each of these segments?

- To what extent do you really tailor the pharmacist's effort to the specific needs and expectations of the segments with which you currently deal?

- What scope exists for focusing in greater detail upon the specifics of these differences and then reflecting this in your marketing effort?

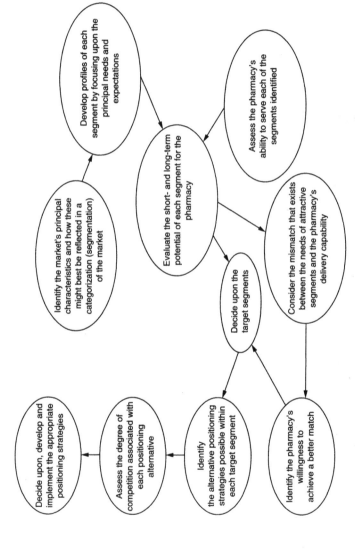

Figure 8.5:   The segmentation, targeting and positioning process

- Which segments appear to offer the greatest future potential?

- What would you need to do in order to target these segments and capitalize upon this potential? Are you/would you be willing to make the investment in staff and facilities that would be needed to do this?

- What positioning stance do you currently adopt? (In thinking about this, give consideration both to the pharmacy's general or overall stance *and* to the specific stance in each of your principal market segments.) What positioning approach might be more appropriate? What would be needed in order to achieve this?

SUMMARY

Within this chapter, we have focused upon the nature and importance of the various elements of the marketing mix and highlighted the need to think about the ways in which the customer list might be segmented and the marketing effort focused more readily.

Because the mix represents the marketing tool kit that is used to shape the profile of the practice and determine the face that is presented to the world, the need to ensure not only that each of the individual elements has been properly developed, but also that they have then been pulled together into a coherent whole is paramount. Any failure to do this is likely to lead to wasted opportunities and a less than optimal performance. However, the reality in many pharmacies is that not only are varying degrees of attention paid to the individual elements, but only rarely is any real attempt also made to pull these together in a truly co-ordinated fashion.

Recognizing this, ask yourself the following questions:

- How frequently do you review in detail each of the individual elements of the mix?

- How clearly stated are the objectives for each element?

- What attention has been paid to the development of an explicit marketing mix action plan?

- To what extent is there a clear strategy for pulling together the individual elements in the form of an integrated and fully co-ordinated marketing programme?

- Who has the overall responsibility for managing the mix?

- How might the customer list be segmented and the marketing effort focused more firmly? What benefits might this lead to?

9

Setting the standards of customer care: the Blackpool rock phenomenon

Having read this chapter, you should:

- understand what contributes to the total customer experience

- appreciate the nature of the interaction between the application of the pharmacist's skills and the staff's skills

- be aware of what would be required of your pharmacy were you to develop an effective customer care programme.

CUSTOMERS ARE PEOPLE TOO

We commented earlier that customers generally take their pharmacist's level of competence for granted and that, because of this, the support elements of the pharmacy are capable of taking on what some pharmacists consider to be an unrealistic or unfair degree of importance in determining not only how the pharmacist is perceived generally, but also how good (or bad) the pharmacy skill dimensions really are. Given this, the argument for focusing upon what we can refer to as the **total customer experience** is inescapable, since it is this that provides the framework for establishing the standards of overall care that customers – your customers – will perceive they are getting from the pharmacist.

There are several reasons why the broader aspects of customer care have increased in importance in recent years, although perhaps the most important and most obvious of these are the generally higher expectations of service that now exist throughout society and an apparent reduction in the willingness of members of the public to make allowances for what they see to be unreasonable behaviour. Couple this with the public's generally greater willingness to complain and take their custom elsewhere, and the arguments for a customer care policy become ever more apparent.

THE BLACKPOOL ROCK PHENOMENON

It needs to be emphasized from the outset that customer care has moved on considerably from the 'have a nice day' – and indeed the 'come back soon, missing you already' – approach that characterized numerous care programmes in the early days. Instead, we are concerned here with establishing the standards that will run right the way through the pharmacy (the Blackpool rock phenomenon), and with achieving the degree of professionalism across the entire spectrum of the framework within which every aspect of pharmacist–customer interaction takes place.

Because of the way in which any truly effective customer care programme for the pharmacist straddles both the pharmacy skills and the support skills dimensions of the pharmacy, you need to begin by considering three fundamental questions.

1. What sort of total experience do you currently give customers? (the reality)

2. What sort of total experience would you like to give? (the intent)

3. What are you really capable of delivering? (the capability)

This reality–intent–capability framework is illustrated in Figure 9.1 and provides a basis for thinking about the size and significance of the gap that exists between intent and capability. There are, of course, numerous factors that can contribute to this gap and having identified its size, significance and the nature of the contributory factors within the pharmacy, thought needs to be given not only to the ways in which the gap might be filled, but also to whether the pharmacist would be willing to allocate the level of resources that would be needed to do this. In making this comment, we have several thoughts in mind, perhaps the most significant of which is that in virtually every pharmacy we have visited, the pharmacist and staff have talked about

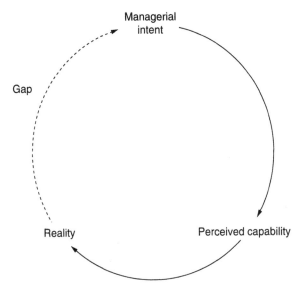

Figure 9.1:   The intent–capability–reality gap

excellence and providing the very highest levels of customer care. The reality, of course, is that what we can refer to as the Rolls Royce approach is only rarely feasible (or cost-effective), and you need therefore to temper your ideas with a dose of reality. To help with this, turn to Figure 9.2 and, being brutally honest with yourself, plot where the pharmacy is currently, and *why*. It might be the case, for example, that you are in Cell Two (high standards of service), but because of antiquated premises, an archaic telephone system and a dragon of an assistant, you have relatively poor levels of support. Having identified the causes in as much detail as possible, you can then begin thinking about what would be required to move the pharmacy either to another cell (presumably Cell One) or to a stronger and more favourable position within the existing cell.

THE LESSONS FROM ELSEWHERE

In our work with a variety of different types of organization, there has proved to be one issue over the past few years that managers have

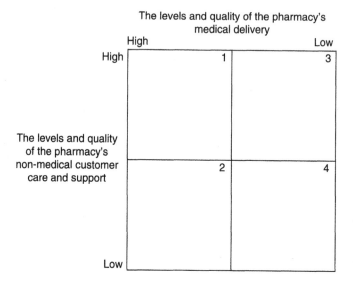

Figure 9.2:   The delivery matrix

discussed with seemingly greater passion than anything else: the standards of customer care and of service that their organizations deliver. Almost without exception, every organization we have dealt with – at least in the first instance – has claimed almost unparalleled levels of customer care, something that has led us to conclude that the business world is full of managers with a seemingly infinite capacity for self-delusion. There are, of course, exceptions to this and it is to these sorts of organization that we now need to turn with a view to learning what it is that contributes to a truly effective customer care programme. However, before doing this, turn to Box 9.1 and think about your experiences in recent weeks as a customer of various types of organization.

Having done this, think about the types of organization that consistently achieve high levels of customer care and about what it is that appears to contribute to this. In the case of the high street, for example, organizations such as Marks & Spencer, Sainsbury and McDonald's have been at the forefront in establishing – and maintaining – the levels of service others simply dream about. In all three cases, the factors that have led to this are straightforward and come down, first, to a fundamental belief on the part of senior management in the importance of customer satisfaction, and then,

Box 9.1:   Your experiences of customer care

Think of three organizations with which you have recently dealt.

- What good and bad experiences do you remember?

- Which of these were related to the behaviour of staff and which to the physical aspects of the place, such as appearance, cleanliness and atmosphere?

- Did there appear to be any real understanding of 'delight' factors (a 'delight' factor is something that makes you feel especially pleased)?

- When you felt that you were treated either badly or less than very well, what was the effect on you?

- Did you bother to complain about the poorish (poor rather than appalling) service or did you simply think that you did not intend helping them to make improvements, and that in future you would go elsewhere?

- When you have been treated badly or less than perfectly, and the organization has been aware of this, what efforts have been made to put things right?

- If you have to go back to a place where you have had a poor experience, what attitudes do you take with you?

- Do you think that your expectations were unreasonable, or would most people react to these experiences in much the same way?

second, to the communication of these values to everyone in the organization. High levels of service – and hence satisfaction – therefore become the norm rather than the exception in these circumstances.

By contrast, the major banks seem to operate according to an altogether completely different set of principles. Instead of being open when customers want (9 am – 6 pm Monday to Saturday and 10 am – 5 pm on Sunday), opening hours reflect staff demands, banking pressures and historical idiosyncrasies. Equally, at the times of highest demand (12 noon – 1.30 pm), staff take lunch breaks and queues form in the branches.

Faced with critical comments such as these, bankers tend to respond by saying, 'But you don't understand our problems'. This sort of response is, however, a nonsense and makes a mockery of any claims of customer service. It is also one of the reasons why the building societies, which have longer opening hours and manage to present a far friendlier face, consistently score far better than the banks in surveys of customer perceptions of care, approachability and friendliness. It is also why telephone banking has been so successful.

The significance of the role played by senior management in these organizations in establishing the standards of service and customer care should never ever be underestimated, something that has been highlighted by the American management guru, Tom Peters. His view is straightforward and unequivocal:

> 'Claims of quality and customer service mean nothing unless the person at the top of the organization is committed to them twenty four hours a day, seven days a week, fifty two weeks a year. If you compromise on this even once, you know it, your staff know it and, worst of all, your customers know it.'

The implications of this for pharmacies, and the need for absolute and total commitment on the part of the staff to the quality of the total customer experience, are (or should be) self-evident.

CUSTOMER CARE IN PHARMACIES

These points were first related to pharmacies in Chapter 3, in which we discussed the customer-oriented pharmacy, and this is not necessarily as difficult as it might appear at first sight. It does, however, involve running the pharmacy for the convenience of the customers rather than, say, the management and staff (this is the equivalent of running the banks for the convenience of the customers rather than the bank staff). In the case of office hours, for example, our experiences have shown that in most instances they were established by the partners themselves several years ago and reflect what is convenient for them rather than what is necessarily the most convenient for their customers. In making this comment, we are not arguing for wholesale changes in how the pharmacy is run but rather for an assessment of whether scope exists for small changes that would prove useful from the customers' point of view. Given this, consider the questions in Box 9.2.

Box 9.2:   The initial customer care audit

- Do those around you *always* behave professionally towards customers and all other members of staff? If not, what problems exist, and *why*?

- What patterns of behaviour do you consider to be unprofessional? What steps have been and are being taken in order to overcome these?

- What do you do if a customer goes away obviously unhappy because of the way in which he has been treated?

- What do you know about the reasons for some customers opting to move to another pharmacy?

In the light of your answers, what picture of the pharmacy do you think emerges and what overall level of customer care do you think the pharmacy manages to achieve?

DEVELOPING A PLAN TO IMPROVE CUSTOMER CARE

Having gone through the initial audit, you can then turn your attention to the ways in which a programme of customer care can be developed. In doing this, you need to follow a simple four-step procedure; this is illustrated in Figure 9.3.

Stage One: The starting point

As a first step, you need to understand in detail how customers currently feel about the pharmacy, what their expectations are, and the extent to which these expectations are not being met. Although you

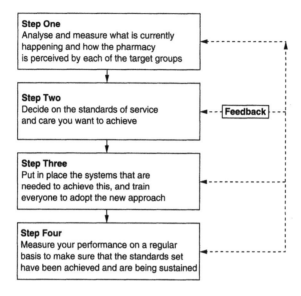

Figure 9.3:   Planning the levels of service and customer care

have already completed the initial audit in Box 9.2, and indeed plotted the position of the pharmacy in Figure 9.2, consider the following additional questions.

- In the light of our comments and questions throughout the book, is the pharmacy fundamentally customer-oriented or pharmacist and staff-oriented?

- Do you really accept that the whole image and physical appearance of the pharmacy is important in contributing to customer care?

- Are you clear about what customers really want from the pharmacy?

- What impression do customers get of the pharmacy when they walk through the door?

- Is it likely that they find any aspect of the pharmacy intimidating or off-putting?

- Do you currently have any formal mechanism that allows customers' views to be fed back and influence how the pharmacy operates?

Stage Two: Setting the standards

Having identified how customers currently perceive the pharmacy, you need then to turn to the question of the overall standards of customer care that you want to aim for. In this, we are assuming that the standards of professional competence are satisfactory. You should therefore focus upon the range of other factors that influence attitudes and performance such as:

- is the pharmacy untidy?
- do the staff appear welcoming and confident?
- is the dispensary clean, modern and efficient?
- does the pharmacist(s) appear welcoming and confident?
- do *all* staff have a good telephone manner and is the phone answered promptly?
- do you make sure that all forms of communication with customers are clear and unambiguous?
- how long do customers normally have to wait for a prescription?
- how accurate is the records system?
- how accessible is the records system?

In the case of your relationships with other stakeholders, such as GPs and nursing homes, think about the answers to the following questions:

- are there opportunities to work more closely with these stakeholders?
- what are you doing to bring this about?
- what changes do you expect to see amongst them over the next two years and the next five years? What are the implications of this?

- who is specifically responsible for ensuring these customers receive good service?

- what information and records do you keep for these customers? What gaps in information do you have?

- what are you doing to set up a system to provide the information to track their business?

Against this background, you can then move on to Stage Three and to the ways in which a customer care programme can be implemented.

Stage Three: Planning and implementing the customer care programme

In planning how to implement a new and higher level of customer care, you need to focus upon five areas:

1.   Developing a customer-oriented pharmacy mission
Make sure that the pharmacy mission statement includes an explicit expression of the level of customer care you are aiming for.

2.   Involving the staff at all stages
Having made a statement of the standards you are aiming for, make sure that staff throughout the pharmacy understand it, believe in it and know how it will be achieved. Make sure that they also feel a sense of ownership. In order to achieve this, ensure that as many staff as possible are involved in deciding what should and needs to be done. There are several ways of doing this, including getting all the staff to complete a questionnaire concerned with what they believe, or know, customers might want from the pharmacy. Other methods for getting ideas involve brainstorming and wide-ranging discussion groups to identify the sorts of change needed.

3.   Defining the requirements of the key activities
For certain key activities define *exactly* what is required and develop procedures to ensure that the activity is carried out in the same way by everyone every time.

4.   Confirm that all staff are part of the customer management process
Customers should know who all staff are – think about putting up a
board with photographs and names so that customers can identify
who is who. The plan also needs to ensure that the role staff play
within the team is continually developed and reinforced, with clear
guidelines being given regarding the limits of their authority.

5.   Staff training
It is essential that all staff are trained to the right level and that
training is continually maintained by the use of refresher courses. In
the case of new staff it is essential that they understand from the
outset what is expected of them. All too often, however, in many
pharmacies the newest member of staff is thrown in at the deep end
and, whilst there are always pressures to make sure that staff are
productive as quickly as possible, any new starter needs to be trained
in the basic procedures before being let loose.

In many cases, the staff who prove most resistant to customer care
training are those who have been in the pharmacy the longest,
believing that they should not be treated as learners along with
the new recruits. However, if you are to achieve a high standard of
customer care across the pharmacy as a whole, all staff need to be
made fully aware of what you are aiming for and what their good and
bad behaviour patterns are. Recognizing this, never compromise by
giving in to individual members of staff and allowing them to miss out
on training sessions. Instead, use them as the basis for team building
as well as developing newly focused customer care skills.

Having gone through the training process, think then about the
ways in which effective performance can be highlighted and rewarded.
One of the easiest and most effective ways of doing this is to ensure
that any favourable comments from customers are passed on or shared
with the relevant staff members. Research consistently emphasizes
the importance of the recognition of achievement as an important
motivator leading to increased job satisfaction and, indirectly, to even
higher levels of customer care.

Stage Four: Measuring the pharmacy's performance

Having set out to develop a customer care programme, you need
to monitor progress and performance on a regular basis. At the

outset, therefore, identify your ten most important customer care dimensions and then measure your performance on these on either a monthly or a quarterly basis. Having acquired this information, you need then to make use of it by feeding back the good and the bad points to everyone in the pharmacy and, where appropriate, identify the changes that need to be made to get back on target.

In the case of retailing, one of the most consistently effective ways of measuring customer care performance has proved to be by means of 'mystery shoppers'. The mystery shopper (MS), who is either an employee from head office or a market researcher, is used by the retailer to explore particular parts of the operation such as the returns policy, the ways in which difficult customers are handled, and the ability of staff to cope with problems at periods of peak demand. The MS therefore goes into the shop, behaves like a customer, and then passes back the details of the experiences, be they good or bad, to head office.

Although we are not making out a case here for mystery customers, there are several lessons that can be learned from this, particularly the need to take an objectively detailed and, in the real sense of the word, naïve look at various parts of the pharmacy from the *customers'* point of view. It is in this way that you can build up a far clearer picture and understanding of what is going right and what is going wrong.

SUMMARY

Within this chapter, we have highlighted the issues that need to be taken into account in developing a customer care programme within the pharmacy. As with many of the initiatives that we have discussed in earlier chapters, you need to identify clearly what your objectives are and then, having determined how these will be achieved, ensure that there is total commitment from across the pharmacy and that the responsibility for driving the programme forward is clearly allocated. Given this, think about the following questions which are then pulled together in the form of a customer care action plan in Box 9.3.

Box 9.3:   The customer care action plan

Our customer care policy is:

The weaknesses in our current approach are:

-
-
-
-
-

To overcome these weaknesses, we need to take action in the following areas:

Action areas   Timescales   Responsibility

-
-
-
-
-
-

The performance measures that will be used to monitor our progress are:

Performance measures   Responsibility

Monthly

-
-
-

Quarterly

-
-
-

Annually

-
-
-

- Do you handle your customers in a way that you can be proud of?

- Do you have a clear and agreed view of the sort of customer care policy that would really be appropriate?

- What is needed in order to implement this?

- Who will take on the responsibility for driving it?

10

Internal marketing, leadership and teamworking: fighting the Napoleonic complex

Having read this chapter, you should:

- understand what is meant by internal marketing

- appreciate the significance of the contribution that internal marketing can make to the effective working of the pharmacy

- recognize the importance of vision, strategy and leadership

- have a greater understanding of what contributes to more effective teams

- appreciate some of the issues associated with effective leadership.

A point that we have made at several stages in this book is that, all too often, plans either falter or fail because of the difficulties associated with their implementation. Recognition of this has led, in recent years, to a considerable amount of attention being paid to the ways in which internal marketing, team building and particular styles of leadership can make the process of implementing a plan both easier and more effective. It is to these three areas that we now turn our attention.

VISION, STRATEGY AND LEADERSHIP

Having worked with a wide variety of organizations over the years, we strongly believe that it is possible to distinguish between good and bad organizations – those that are effective and those that are

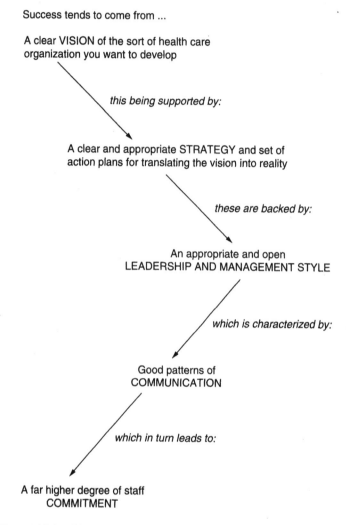

Success tends to come from ...

A clear VISION of the sort of health care
organization you want to develop

this being supported by:

A clear and appropriate STRATEGY and set of
action plans for translating the vision into reality

these are backed by:

An appropriate and open
LEADERSHIP AND MANAGEMENT STYLE

which is characterized by:

Good patterns of
COMMUNICATION

which in turn leads to:

A far higher degree of staff
COMMITMENT

Figure 10.1:   Vision, strategy and leadership

ineffective – by examining them against the background of the
deceptively simple model that is illustrated in Figure 10.1.

The thinking behind the model is straightforward. If an organization, regardless of its type or size, is to move ahead effectively, it
is essential that those running it have a clear *vision* of the sort of

organization they are trying to develop; that there is a clear *strategy* and set of action plans for achieving this; and that a clear and appropriate *leadership/management* style exists. These are then reinforced by open patterns of *communication* so that the staff are fully aware of the direction in which the organization is going, what is expected of them and how they will benefit. Given this, *levels of commitment* are likely to increase substantially.

In the light of this model, there are several questions that you need to consider; these appear in Box 10.1.

Box 10.1:   The vision, strategy, leadership and communication checklist

The vision

- How clear a vision exists of the sort of pharmacy that you and your team are trying to develop? (In answering this, you might refer back to our discussion of the importance of vision in Chapter 6.)

- To what extent is this vision clouded by either disharmony between the staff or a failure to discuss it in detail?

- Given your location, resources and any other constraints, how realistic is this vision?

- How effectively has this vision been communicated to staff?

The strategy and action plan

- How well thought out are the action plans?

- How explicit are they?

- How well resourced are they?

- How well have patterns of responsibility been allocated?

The leadership/management styles

- What sort of leadership/management styles exist within the pharmacy

- How appropriate are these styles, given the staff that you have and the anticipated demands of the late 20th and early 21st centuries?

continued

Box 10.1: *continued*

- How do the staff perceive these styles?
- What evidence is there of dissatisfaction with them?

Communication

- How well developed are the patterns of communication within the pharmacy?
- Does information flow in all directions?
- What obstacles to good information flow exist?
- What communication-related problems have been encountered?

We have quite deliberately not asked any questions in Box 10.1 about levels of commitment, since it should be apparent by now that the commitment of staff will be influenced to a very substantial degree by the leadership/management styles and patterns of communication that exist. However, before going any further and discussing how levels of commitment might be increased by internal marketing, it is worth taking a step sideways and looking at the work in the 1950s of Douglas McGregor, in particular his development of Theory X and Theory Y. In essence, McGregor argues that there are few inherently bad employees, but plenty of bad managers. People, he suggests, typically have the capacity for self-motivation and, in general, it is management styles and organizational structures and constraints that inhibit this and prevent people making a worthwhile contribution; these ideas are summarized in Box 10.2.

It follows from this, and indeed from the earlier part of the chapter, that the pharmacy is likely to work in a far more effective manner if certain broad guidelines are adhered to. An important starting point in this is the development of open patterns of communication, with staff being kept fully aware of how the organization is developing. Two immediately valuable tools for this are internal marketing and the development of teams. However, before looking at these two areas, ask yourself which of McGregor's two theories most closely typifies ways of thinking within the pharmacy?

Box 10.2:   McGregor's Theory X and Theory Y

Working in the 1950s, McGregor identified two patterns of thought and assumptions about people in organizations.

Theory X argues that people are:

- inherently lazy and work as little as possible

- lacking in ambition, dislike responsibility and prefer to be led

- self-centred, indifferent to organizational needs, and resistant to change

- gullible and not very bright.

By contrast, Theory Y suggests that people:

- are not by nature passive or resistant to organizational needs, but have become so as the result of their experiences in organizations

- have an enormous capacity for motivation, development and responsibility, and that structures and systems need to be designed to reflect this and reduce the constraints and levels of control.

SO WHAT IS INTERNAL MARKETING?

The idea of internal marketing is straightforward and is based on the idea that an organization will operate far more effectively if its staff have a clear understanding of core values and objectives and are able to identify with these. To achieve this empathy, there is a need to recruit appropriate people, give them a strong sense of identity and operating freedom, and support them with good patterns of communication and open management styles. Assuming this is done properly, the pay-offs can be considerable and are likely to be reflected in far higher levels of motivation and commitment. (These ideas were first touched upon in our discussion in Chapter 1 of the 7-S framework.)

In the light of these comments, consider the questions that appear below:

- Do the staff really understand the pharmacy's core values and objectives and empathize with them?

- Do you feel that you really have the right type and blend of staff within the pharmacy?

- Do you spend enough time training staff and equipping them with the necessary skills?

- How often are problems caused by poor communications?

- Do your staff feel that they have sufficient operating freedom?

- Are the patterns of communication sufficiently open?

- How involved are your staff in deciding how the pharmacy is run?

Against the background of your answers to these questions, think about the leadership styles that exist within the pharmacy (these are discussed again at a later stage in this chapter in Box 10.4 and Figure 10.2). Are they, for example, essentially a reflection of a 'tells' approach in which having made a decision, you and your colleagues simply tell the staff what to do, or is it rather more of a 'sells' style, in which you sell the idea to others by discussing it in some detail and giving consideration to the implications for them? Another possible approach is the consultative style, in which you only make the decision after having discussed the various aspects with those who are involved or who are likely to be affected. Internal marketing gives full recognition to the need to carry staff with you and therefore to the crucial importance of making sure that patterns of com- munication are as open as possible and that staff feel a strong sense of involvement. Without this, it is likely that you are simply failing to exploit the real potential of the pharmacy and the people in it.

THE ROLE OF TEAMS

As part of the overall process of internal marketing and improving pharmacy effectiveness, you need to give explicit consideration to the scope that exists for teamworking and to the nature of any blocks to teamworking that currently exist. In doing this, you need to recognize that every member of staff is, or should be, capable of making a direct or indirect contribution to customer satisfaction. Recognition of this highlights the crucial importance of teams and teamworking throughout the pharmacy.

THE PROS AND CONS OF TEAMWORKING

The benefits that can come from teamworking can be substantial and include:

- the support that colleagues can give to individuals so that they can more easily develop and exploit their strengths

- the ways in which teams can build upon the different ideas and skills that individual members of the team possess

- the ways in which the team can capitalize upon the previous experiences of staff in doing a similar job in different circumstances

- the discovery of particular skills that in normal circumstances might be hidden, but that frequently emerge when teamworking

- the ways in which, by ensuring staff familiarize themselves with colleagues' jobs, the pharmacy can avoid an overdependence on individuals, reduce the load on some staff members at times of crisis, and reduce the risk of procedures being carried out differently and incorrectly

- ensuring that customers can gain from a better 'experience' in a visit to the pharmacy through a more highly co-ordinated approach

- a sense of shared purpose and the general levels of synergy that teams can achieve.

There are, of course, some potential dangers of teamworking that can cause problems:

- It can expose the weaknesses of some members of staff and reinforce the egos and positions of those members of staff who see themselves as 'experts'.

- To be successful, teamworking requires staff to alternate between leading, supporting and perhaps being on the sidelines at different times, and this continual change in relationships can prove difficult for some staff to handle.

On balance, however, the pros of teamwork outweigh any possible cons by a substantial margin. Recognizing this, the question that needs to be considered is how more effective teams can be developed within the pharmacy.

BUILDING MORE EFFECTIVE TEAMS

Only rarely, if ever, is there an opportunity to build a team from scratch and, in many pharmacies, there are relatively infrequent opportunities even to modify teams other than at the margin when, for example, someone leaves and someone new is brought in. It is possible, however, to make adjustments by controlling some members of staff, encouraging others in a certain direction and, when recruiting, doing it with a deep-seated understanding of the balances and imbalances that currently exist within different parts of the pharmacy. Questions that can help in this by providing a greater insight into your existing teams appear in Box 10.3. Remember, therefore, that when forming or building a team, you need to aim for a blend of strengths, skills and personalities, and should avoid creating one that simply reinforces the status quo.

SO WHAT CONTRIBUTES TO MORE EFFECTIVE TEAMS?

The guidelines for building more effective teams are relatively straightforward and include:

- ensuring that the team has a distinct and measurable purpose

- providing constructive feedback on performance

- varying the team's tasks and responsibilities over time

- rotating staff on a periodic and planned basis so that new talents and ideas are injected into the team and so that the membership and patterns of thinking do not become too incestuous or complacent

- gradually increasing the degree of autonomy

- encouraging the team to redefine their responsibilities and tasks.

Box 10.3: The teamworking checklist

- What teams do you currently have within the pharmacy?

- Do you make as much use of teams as you might?

- How well do your teams currently work?

- What obstacles to better teamworking exist?

- Do you have well-balanced teams, or do they appear to be dominated by particular individuals?

- What changes would be needed in order to achieve a better balance of skills?

- Do the members of the teams appear to have sufficiently complementary skills?

- What appear to be the current attitudes and levels of motivation of various team members? Do they need to be modified in any way? (Do not assume that good working relationships automatically lead to effectiveness. Indeed, they can lead to a degree of complacency in which old working practices and conventional wisdoms are never challenged or changed for the better.)

- How are junior staff treated, and what roles do they appear to be playing within the teams? Are they simply being tolerated, or are real efforts being made by other team members to use their skills and develop their abilities?

Against the background of these comments, consider the following questions:

- do you trust the members of your team?

- do they trust you?

- is there mutual trust?

- do you respect the members of your team?

- do they respect you?

- is there mutual respect?

- is the atmosphere open and supportive?

- can you handle success and failure?

- are workloads properly balanced?

- are the team members loyal to you and/or to the pharmacy and to each other?

- is the team mutually supportive?

- can you and other team members express true opinions?

- do you plan, organize, review and communicate effectively?

- does everyone feel part of the team?

- does each team have a clear sense of direction?

ASPECTS OF LEADERSHIP

In 1996, we carried out a study amongst a number of professionals, including solicitors, doctors, pharmacists and accountants. In doing this, we were attempting to find out how professionals are viewed by their key staff. The findings led us to suggest that 'the average professional is a poor manager who has appalling communication skills, little real idea of how to plan, fewer ideas of how to motivate staff, and typically adopts an inconsistent and idiosyncratic style of management and leadership'.

These conclusions need to be seen against the general background of the work, in which we examined the principal roles that pharmacists are typically expected to perform:

- a *professional carer or adviser* role

- a *leadership* role

- a *team building* and *team player* role

Although the majority of the staff surveyed seemed to feel that the professional adviser role is carried through fairly well, they proved to be far less complimentary about the extent to which the leadership and team roles were either recognized or performed. It was this that then led us to categorize the professionals along the two dimensions that we introduced earlier: their *willingness* to manage and their *ability* to manage.

Balancing the three roles: the problems of leadership

Although our research showed that the pharmacist's technical skills were generally (but not invariably) acknowledged by their staff, an all too common feeling among staff appeared to be that they used this as an excuse for both their appalling leadership and teamworking skills, and for the ways in which staff were all too frequently expected to operate with a degree of telepathy.

With regard to the *leadership* role, our work suggested that interpretations of how best to fulfil this appear to vary enormously. For some, leadership appears to mean giving orders and just telling the staff what to do, with little or no real attempt being made to explain why or how; it was this that led us to suggest that in a surprisingly high number of instances there appeared to be a need to fight the Napoleonic complex. For others, but seemingly a minority, leadership proved to be a far more meaningful activity which involved developing strong and effective communication networks, giving emphasis to staff development, and ensuring that everyone understood what was expected of them. For yet others, it was something in which they showed a vague, if amateurish, interest every now and again (generally when they did not appear to have much else to do).

A further area that led to problems of leadership was what we labelled the closed file syndrome, with the staff being denied access to areas of information – particularly financial – and excluded from any involvement in important decisions. Instead, they were simply told the outcome of a planning meeting and then expected to show great enthusiasm and commitment to the process of implementation. Given these comments, turn to Box 10.4 and think about the sort of overall style that you exhibit.

Box 10.4:   Leadership styles

- The PROPHET has a vision

- The BARBARIAN is pragmatic, forceful and action-oriented

- The BUILDER develops structures

- The EXPLORER develops skills

- The SYNERGIST balances skills and structures

- The ADMINISTRATOR integrates systems to achieve perfect financial control and management within the pharmacy

- The BUREAUCRAT applies tight controls, cuts costs and has no desire to be creative

- The ARISTOCRAT inherits, does no work but upsets the team

What does your response tell you about yourself?

BUILDING AND MOTIVATING THE PHARMACY'S TEAMS

The third area we looked at in the research was the teamworking role and, in particular, how it was interpreted. All too often, there was a failure to recognize the extent of the contribution that was needed, or indeed the considerable amount of time and effort involved in building, developing and maintaining effective teams. Instead, it appeared frequently to be believed either that teams would emerge as if by magic or that the sole responsibility for team building rested with others.

These problems were then exacerbated by the ways in which some pharmacists automatically blamed staff for lost letters or records and rarely – if ever – admitted to their mistakes.

When it came to motivation, pharmacists appeared to perform equally badly by working on the basis that staff should not worry because they would be told when they got it wrong. (Good staff, it is commonly believed, never need their egos massaging by being told when they get things right!)

THE NINE DEADLY SINS

Typical of the other managerial mistakes made that were highlighted by the study were:

- the failure to recognize that staff have work schedules and need holidays and cannot necessarily always take on extra jobs, or work late on extra days

- making decisions for their own benefit without thinking of the consequences for others

- not agreeing the boundaries of staff responsibility and authority

- working on a need-to-know basis

- persisting with poor communication networks so that mistakes are repeated

- taking a 'don't bother me, I'm too busy' attitude

- breaking the rules and undermining the guidelines laid down for the pharmacy

- not knowing enough about individual members of staff, their aspirations, motivations and limitations

- operating unnecessary and bureaucratic procedures for no real purpose.

Although we know that none of these criticisms can be levelled at *you*, as the reader, you might find it useful to take each of the points in turn and think about the extent to which others within your pharmacy are guilty of these sorts of mistakes. Having done this, think about the consequences for the staff and, in particular, for levels of motivation, morale and team effectiveness.

SUMMARY: SO WHAT ARE THE IMPLICATIONS OF THIS?

We started off this chapter by suggesting that the successful implementation of plans is often hampered by certain styles of leadership and poorly developed and badly managed teams, two elements that highlight the need for a programme of internal as well as external marketing. Recognizing this, think about how, if at all, internal marketing is currently manifested within the pharmacy and how an internal marketing programme might possibly be either developed or improved. As part of this, give thought also to the nature of the teamworking and leadership styles that exist and to the scope that exists for their development and improvement. In the case of leadership styles, Figure 10.2 provides a framework for categorizing the predominant style. Given that a participative style is arguably the most appropriate for a professional organization such as a pharmacy, you might like to consider whether you appear to have the right mix and, if not, the sorts of problem this creates and what would be involved in changing the balance.

The final issue that you need to consider at this stage is the extent to which you pay attention to internal marketing and how this might be improved. To help with this, you might go back to the questions that we posed earlier in the chapter in our explanation of what internal marketing involves, and then consider how you perform in terms of what we refer to as 'the door exercise'. This is a straightforward concept, based on the idea that, like a door, management

| | The extent of management authority | |
	High	Low
High	**Consultative** Managers discuss the decision with others who might be involved. Having listened to these views, the manager then makes the decision	**Participative** The manager discusses the decision with others who are involved, and they then take the decision jointly
Staff freedom and involvement in decision-making		
	Autocratic The manager simply makes all the decisions and tells the staff what they have to do	**Paternalistic** The manager makes the decision and then 'sells' this to those who are affected, so that they understand it and will implement it with a degree of enthusiasm
Low		

Figure 10.2: The four leadership styles

styles can be opened, closed or ajar. In the case of the open door styles, staff make regular and significant contributions to the development of the pharmacy, because they know:

- how the pharmacy works

- what is expected of them in terms of daily routines

- that they are encouraged to put forward their ideas

- how their ideas and suggestions will be evaluated and used

- what the future aims and objectives of the pharmacy are and how they can best contribute

- that they would be involved if painful decisions had to be made, so that the outcome would not come as a bolt out of the blue.

In pharmacies where the door is partially open, staff are kept informed on an irregular basis, influenced as much by crises and mistakes as anything else. Other stimuli are the pharmacist reading a book advocating open communication and needing the staff to rally round when problems arise.

In many ways, this is the worst situation for staff as they never really know where they stand. One day they feel motivated and enthusiastic because their contributions have been asked for and recognized, whilst the next day they will feel ignored and insignificant. In this situation, staff are often expected to offer instant solutions to problems when crises occur, but are not expected to contribute to planning for longer-term improvements, never really know if their unsolicited contributions will be welcome or scorned and do not really know what is expected of them.

Where the door is fully closed, the managers make every decision themselves and let staff have the minimum information that they need simply to perform their tasks.

The staff in this situation are very clear about their role and what is expected of them. For some, particularly those who have no real commitment to the pharmacy, their job is simply a way of earning a salary until they find something better. For others who look for more from a job, the experience is extraordinarily frustrating. These staff frequently feel resentful when their intelligence is insulted and their self-respect damaged. The pharmacist makes it obvious that they have the responsibility for many aspects of the pharmacy and as the complexity of running pharmacies increases, more and more problems emerge. In these circumstances, staff become increasingly resentful and retreat so that they will not look for things that are going wrong and may even feel some satisfaction when a crisis occurs and the pharmacist makes a mistake.

11

Implementing the plan and making things happen

Having read this chapter, you should:

- understand more clearly the nature and cause of the factors that help or hinder the development and implementation of marketing plans

- have a greater insight into the ways in which obstacles might possibly be overcome

- have developed a framework for implementing a marketing programme for your pharmacy.

Throughout this book, we have concentrated upon developing a relatively pragmatic approach reflecting an emphasis on the issues that are associated with the development and implementation of a stronger customer-centred approach to the marketing of pharmacies. Within this chapter, we pull some of these ideas together in the form of an action plan that should provide the framework for your pharmacy's future marketing effort.

THE BARRIERS TO IMPLEMENTATION

We have already made the observation that planning is generally a relatively straightforward activity, but that plans too often founder during their implementation phase. Although there are numerous reasons for this, the most common have proved to be over-ambitious objectives, unrealistic timescales, inadequate funding, a lack of staff (and pharmacist) commitment and/or feeling of ownership concerning its implementation, and, perhaps most importantly, the absence of someone with sufficient authority who is willing to take on the responsibility for driving the plan on a day-to-day basis. Given these points, consider the following questions:

- Are you at all guilty of setting objectives that, whilst they look impressive, are likely to prove too ambitious? (The hopeless optimism phenomenon.)

- Are you trying to do too much in too short a time?

- Have you really thought through the funding implications of the plan and are you confident that funding will not be a problem?

- Are you likely to experience any skills shortages during the period covered by the plan?

- Have you made sure that staff throughout the pharmacy have been involved in the planning process, kept informed of what you are setting out to achieve, and are fully committed to the plan?

- Have you allocated responsibilities properly?

- Do you have the right person to drive the plan forward (the plan's 'champion')?

- Have you built in the appropriate checks?

- Have you scheduled a series of planning review meetings to monitor progress?

- Have you given sufficient thought to the factors that might make the implementation of the plan easier and/or more effective?

Assuming that you are satisfied with the answers to these questions, you can then turn your attention to the action planning framework that is illustrated in Box 11.1. All that remains for us is to wish you happy (and successful) marketing planning!

In a majority of pharmacies, however, the planning and implementation process often proves to be a rather more difficult exercise. Given this, turn to Figure 11.1, which is designed to highlight the sorts of implementation problems that you might possibly encounter.

Box 11.1: The marketing action-planning framework

Marketing objectives (in order) of priority)	Actions required	Timing	Costs	Responsibility	Interim performance measures
•					
•					
•					
•					
•					
•					
•					
•					
•					
•					

Having worked your way through the diagram, it should be apparent that there are several major potential problem areas. These include:

- failing to take sufficient account of the environment

- overestimating what the pharmacy is really capable of delivering

- failing to recognize the real significance of staff commitment and of the need for a sense of staff ownership of the plan

- assuming that implementation will take place even though the specific responsibility for driving the plan has not been clearly allocated

- failing to recognize that even the very best plans may encounter problems or need modifying as the result of an unpredictable shift in the environment.

Recognition of these issues leads fairly logically to the ideas and process encapsulated in Figure 11.2.

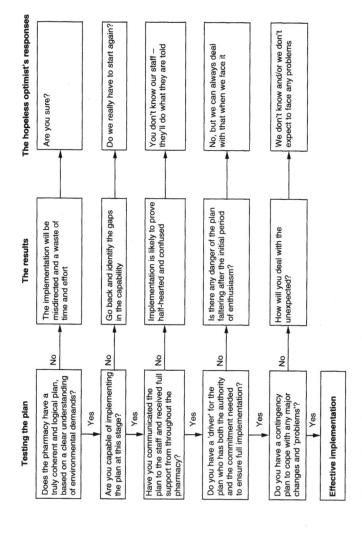

Figure 11.1: Identifying possible implementation problems

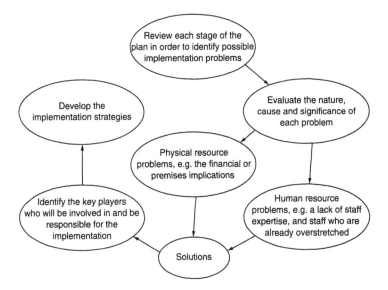

Figure 11.2: Dealing with implementation problems

SUMMARY

Come to the Edge
We might fall
Come to the Edge
It's too high!
COME TO THE EDGE
And they came
and he pushed
and they flew.

Index

9 781857 752021